Functional Anatomy

of the

Pilates Core

An Illustrated Guide to a Safe and Effective Core Training Program

Evan Osar and Marylee Bussard

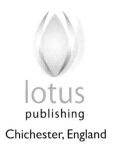

lotus
publishing

Chichester, England

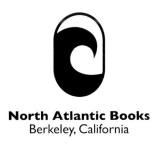

North Atlantic Books
Berkeley, California

First published in 2015 by
Lotus Publishing
Apple Tree Cottage, Inlands Road, Nutbourne, Chichester, PO18 8RJ and
North Atlantic Books
Berkeley, California

Drawings Amanda Williams
Text Design Mary-Anne Trant
Cover Design Paula Morrison
Printed and Bound in Malaysia by Tien Wah Press

MEDICAL DISCLAIMER: The following information is intended for general information purposes only. Individuals should always see their health care provider before administering any suggestions made in this book. Any application of the material set forth in the following pages is at the reader's discretion and is his or her sole responsibility.

Functional Anatomy of the Pilates Core: An Illustrated Guide to a Safe and Effective Core Training Program is sponsored and published by the Society for the Study of Native Arts and Sciences (dba North Atlantic Books), an educational nonprofit based in Berkeley, California, that collaborates with partners to develop cross-cultural perspectives, nurture holistic views of art, science, the humanities, and healing, and seed personal and global transformation by publishing work on the relationship of body, spirit, and nature.

North Atlantic Books' publications are available through most bookstores. For further information, visit our website at www.northatlanticbooks.com or call 800-733-3000.

British Library Cataloguing-in-Publication Data
A CIP record for this book is available from the British Library
ISBN 978 1 905367 55 9 (Lotus Publishing)
ISBN 978 1 58394 999 3 (North Atlantic Books)

Library of Congress Cataloguing-in-Publication Data
Osar, Evan, 1969-
  Functional anatomy of the pilates core : an illustrated guide to a safe and effective core training program / Evan Osar and Marylee Bussard.
    pages cm
  ISBN 978-1-58394-999-3 (paperback) — ISBN 978-1-62317-002-8 (ebook)
  1. Pilates method. 2. Body movement. 3. Mind and body. I. Bussard, Marylee. II. Title.
  RA781.4.O83 2016
  613.7'192—dc23
                                    2015013340

Contents

To all our patients and clients: The strategies in this book have been developed through our work together and because of the trust each of you places in us. Thank you for taking this journey with us and for allowing us the opportunity to serve you.

Acknowledgments

I would like to thank the publisher, Jon Hutchings of Lotus Publishing, for providing me with the opportunity and the creative freedom to write this book with Marylee. Jon is one of the kindest and most patient individuals in the industry and possibly the best publisher an author could work with.

A special thank you goes to all the incredible leaders of the rehabilitation and fitness industries who have influenced my career. This extensive list includes, but is not limited to, Paul Hodges, Vladimir Janda, Gwendolyn Jull, Pavel Kolář, Diane Lee, Linda Joy Lee, Karel Lewit, and Shirley Sahrmann. You will see their influences throughout this book.

And of course Joseph Pilates, one of the pioneers of the movement industry, deserves a special mention. As I began research for this book I was struck by how much overlap there was between our current concepts in core conditioning and Pilates' original teaching. It is my hope that this book builds upon his concepts and will be a valuable resource for the industry.

Finally, to my beautiful wife Jenice: You empower me every single day to be the best I can be and to serve with confidence, humility, and integrity. I am blessed every day because you are part of my life. This world is a better place because you are in it.

Photographer: Jon Eatinger

Photo credits: Fred Miller, Pierre Cameron

Models: Marylee Bussard, Ellen Letten, Marcy Schlessinger, Evan Osar, Melissa Posh, Natalie Rothgreb, A.J. Taylor-Vanderpool

Evan Osar

www.fitnesseducationseminars.com

I would like to thank all of my outstanding bodywork teachers and sources of inspiration, especially Evan Osar, Tom Myers, Lou Benson, Andrew Mannino, Larry Phipps, Kelly Chadwick, James Earls, Robert Schliep and Divo Muller, Doug and Alicia Zabrocki, Shirley Sahrman, Ida Rolf, Janet Travell, Karen Clippinger, Gray Cook, Eric Franklin, Blandine Calais-Germain, Michael Eastwood, and Anat Baniel.

A special thank you goes to all of my colleagues, clients, and advisors at Chaturanga Fitness, who have supported me on this path and taught me so much! Thank you to Laura Coe, in particular, who taught me how nurturing the deep core is a lesson not just for the body, but for our business and personal lives too.

Finally, I extend my deepest gratitude to my grandmother, my mother, and my Aunt Loretta for always being there for me; to my big sister, Tiffany, for being the first person to tell me about this exercise called Pilates; and to my precious home-base, the ever-loving Chris and Jake Smoot. Chris, you bring balance and clarity to my life just as you do for the water systems you restore in your work. Thank you for making all of this possible.

Marylee Bussard

www.chaturangafitness.com

Abbreviations

ANS	autonomic nervous system
ASIS	anterior superior iliac spine
BAS	Breath Activation Strategy
CNS	central nervous system
DMS	deep myofascial system
FAI	femoroacetabular impingement
GERD	gastroesophageal reflux disease
GI	gastrointestinal
HIIT	high-intensity interval training
IAP	intra-abdominal pressure
ITB	iliotibial band
KI	kinesthetic intelligence
PMA	Pilates Method Alliance
PNS	peripheral nervous system (can also stand for parasympathetic nervous system)
SIJ	sacroiliac joint
SMFR	self-myofascial release
SMS	superficial myofascial system
SNS	somatic nervous system
TFL	tensor fasciae latae
TL	thoracolumbar
TLJ	thoracolumbar junction
TPC	thoracopelvic canister
TVA	transversus abdominis

Introduction to the Pilates Principles

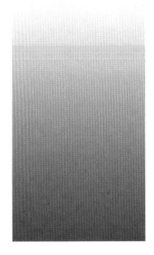

1

"Why boast of this age of science and invention that has produced so many marvelous wonders when, in the final analysis, we find that man has in the race for material progress and perfection, entirely overlooked the most complex and marvelous of all Creations—Man himself!"

J.H. Pilates in *Your Health*, 1934

By the time he wrote these words, Joseph Pilates was fifty years old. He was living in New York City at the height of the Great Depression, having left behind his native Europe during the short peace between two world wars. His life also corresponded with an unparalleled pace of discovery and invention that utterly transformed civilization, in the form of the automobile, airplanes, color photography, sound movies, radio, television, penicillin, and the theory of relativity. For all the rapid change and upheaval of the early twentieth century, Pilates could scarcely have imagined the "marvelous wonders" that were waiting for humanity, just around the corner. And yet, in today's Internet Age, Joseph Pilates' call to remember the body, "the most complex and marvelous of all Creations," resonates across the decades with more relevance to people living today than ever before. Why boast of all

our accomplishments, wrote Pilates, when we have lost touch with our very own bodies? Our bodies, organic and receptive, have adapted to changing work and home environments, deferentially molding themselves to the technology upon which we have come to rely. This trend is famously captured in the cartoon that charts man's evolution from primate to bipedal hominid, to early human hunter, to modern slouching desk worker. An unfortunate by-product of our "race for material progress and perfection," in other words, seems to be a profusion of humans with chair-shaped spines.

Against civilization's overwhelming historical march towards "progress," Joseph Pilates stood—with his strange machines fashioned from reconfigured wheelchairs, bedframes, and beer kegs—to re-enliven humanity, as do we who carry forward his work today. The son of a gymnast and a naturopath, Pilates put forth a model for physical life that enabled modern people to reconnect with their natural somatic instincts. It is said that, as a child, Pilates spent long hours in the woods watching animals, and that the movements of stray cats provided inspiration for him during his wartime internment on the Isle of Man, where the early seeds of what we now know as Pilates took root in his mind.

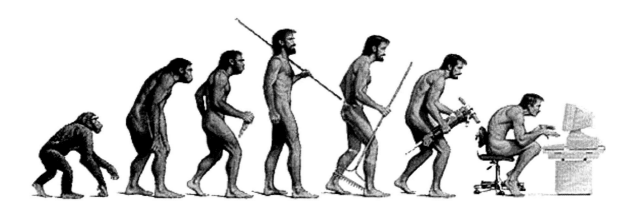

Figure 1.1: Evolution from primate to bipedal hominid, to early human hunter, to modern slouching desk worker.

Eventually, he brought these keenly developed powers of observation across the Atlantic to bear upon the deteriorated physical state of his fellow urban dwellers in New York. He criticized the "brutalizing training regimens" and "artificial exercise" widely considered to be the path to health but which seemed to him to disregard scientific and functional principles. He decried the misguided ways in which children's innate physical intelligence was stifled by adults, "whose physical and mental balance was either deranged or, perhaps, never even attained." Perhaps it is no coincidence that back pain is now the leading cause of disability globally, stifling productivity and enjoyment of life for countless numbers of otherwise prosperous people of *all* ages.

My (Marylee's) grandmother was a little girl living in New York at the time Pilates wrote these words. Two generations later, I watched helplessly as failed back surgery after failed back surgery robbed her of vitality. With all of technology's promise of a more connected world and a better quality of life, no quick-fix device or innovation has emerged in the past century to reverse the growing incidence of age- and lifestyle-related spinal disorders. It is common to assume that these kinds of degenerative change are just an inevitable part of the aging process, but I think Pilates was on to something. If everyone could find a way to restore what was stifled and eventually lost in the children Pilates observed, then maybe we could rewrite our own twenty-first century endings and remain active and pain-free until our final days.

The Lost Wisdom of Kinesthesia

It has been said that you cannot outsource exercising; in other words, no one can do it for you. We would add that you cannot "tune out" truly functional exercise. Today, many exercise programs emphasize fast pace and high intensity, in the hopes that we can squeeze more benefit into shorter workouts. Like the "brutalizing training regimens" Pilates described in the early twentieth century, for the average person such workouts leave little room for *subtlety, centering, precision, curiosity,* and awareness—all principles that awaken the "innate physical intelligence" to which Joe was referring.

Fortunately, more and more personal trainers, physical therapists, and body workers are beginning to grasp the importance of kinesthetic awareness—how our body moves and the ability to be "present" in our body and aware of its sensations. Without kinesthetic intelligence, we are disconnected from our bodies; we miss out on the physical dance of life, and many of the body's countless daily requests to adjust, stretch, and express itself physically are tuned out, making us more prone to stiffness, pain, injury, and degenerative changes. Science is beginning to support the notion that the *quality of our attention* can have transforming effects on all systems of the body: neurological, circulatory, respiratory, visceral, psycho-emotional, energetic, and myofascial. Slowing down and paying attention so that kinesthetic awareness can awaken is—or at least, ought to be—the very essence of the rehabilitative process.

The great news is that holistic fitness programs like yoga and Pilates are now widespread. From enlightened Baby Boomers who suffered overuse injuries during the "no pain, no gain" fitness days of the '80s and '90s, to college and pro sports teams, people who need a sustainable exercise strategy are looking to us. This growing trend foretells a shift, not just in the nature and content of our workouts, but also in the role of exercise itself as an indispensable piece of the healthcare continuum. With a growing aging population and lifestyle diseases such as diabetes, heart disease, and osteoporosis on the rise, the general population requires sensible exercise choices that nurture functional strength and awareness in preference to punishing routines and unrealistic goals.

Pilates instructors are uniquely positioned to lead the way in this holistic fitness revolution. Whether your Pilates training is "classical" or "evolved," Pilates is, and always has been, a corrective exercise program at its core, conceived and designed to restore modern (wo)man to a more optimal alignment and more efficient patterns of movement. During the past fifteen years in particular, practitioners from diverse disciplines—including dance, gymnastics, yoga, Feldenkrais, manual therapies, personal training, sports medicine, and physical therapy—have added new dimensions to the work of Joseph Pilates. With this book, we bring together ideas from these various fields to help ensure that this century-old program remains as relevant and beneficial today as it was in Pilates' time. We also hope that Pilates teachers and enthusiasts will gain a better understanding of the "complex and marvelous … Creation" that we are. May the ideas explored here help you further Joe's wish to enliven body, mind, and spirit and awaken you to your true nature.

Pilates for the Twenty-first Century

While considerable diversity exists in the ways that Pilates is practiced and taught today, six principles derived from Joseph Pilates' writings are widely accepted and cited in the Pilates community as the defining features of this exercise system. They are as follows: Centering, Concentration, Control, Precision, Breath, and Flow. Let's look at each of the six principles of Pilates through a modern lens. In particular, we will consider how these excellent foundational guidelines are reinforced and complemented by principles emerging out of recent discoveries in two dynamic fields of research: neuroplasticity and fascia.

Neuroplasticity is the brain's ability to reorganize itself by developing new neuronal connections. It was once believed that this ability of the brain to change itself was limited after a certain age, but in recent years discoveries have revealed that the brain is learning and changing throughout one's lifespan. We can leverage the brain's plasticity to create the changes we want to see in our lives, including our bodies.

The lessons of neuroplasticity suggest that practicing Pilates can be much more than executing graceful choreography to strengthen and elongate the muscles of the body. Pilates can also be a vehicle for creating a vibrant mind. Like food for the nervous system, curious and attentive states of mind attract new neuronal activity. Sensory nerves swim like fishes to those areas where our attention summons them, and in a Pilates session that can mean an oceanful of kinesthetic "swimming" and brain rewiring.

Being playful, interested, and exploratory in our routines and cueing fosters greater mental and physical dexterity. As we practice new skills and master subtle changes, we notice and concentrate, try and fail, adapt and try again. Through this process, function improves, not necessarily because we will it to, but because the body discovers more-efficient options it previously did not know that it had. By this logic, Pilates is not only about precisely executing exercises; it is about exploring and adapting them in order to create new options for the body.

Fascia refers to the connective tissues of the body, including the alternately viscous, tough fibrous, and delicate web-like matrix within which everything inside the body floats. Previously considered to be mere "packing material" for the cells and organs of the body, fascia is now understood to be involved in much more. Because of its dense innervation with mechanoreceptors, fascia's role includes sensing and adapting to the mechanical forces placed upon the body. For example, wherever continuous loading occurs, the fascia reorganizes itself by thickening in response to the greater demand placed upon it. Most sports injuries relate to connective tissue (fascia) as opposed to muscles or bones, and increasing numbers of sports teams are beginning to incorporate exercises (like Pilates and Yoga) that improve fascial elasticity and resiliency.

There is also an important perceptual dimension to fascial training and fascial injury prevention, which we will discuss next.

Exercising the Neuromyofascial System

In fact, the brain/nervous system and the muscle and fascial systems are intimately intertwined. Pioneers in the developing field of exercise known as *fascial fitness* (Robert Schliep, Divo Muller, and Tom Myers), as well as specialists focused on improving brain function through movement and exercise (such as Anat Baniel, who is a protégé of Moshe Feldenkrais and works with adults and children with developmental and cognitive impairments), offer scientifically grounded insights into improving function in what many are now referring to as the *neuromyofascial system*. In the next section, we will explore how these discoveries can transform your Pilates practice.

The Six Pilates Principles (Reimagined)

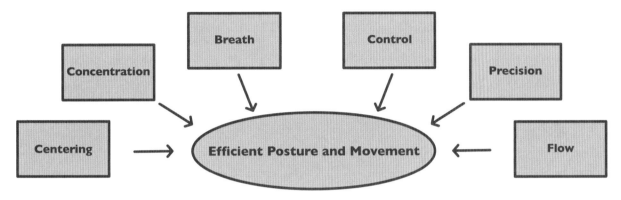

Figure 1.2: The six Pilates principles (reimagined).

I. Centering

The principle of **Centering** is Pilates' *defining characteristic*. This principle reflects Joseph Pilates' understanding that all movement begins and emanates from the center. The center of gravity of the body lies in front of the sacrum, about three finger-widths below the navel (this is known as the *lower dantian* in martial arts). As we move through our daily activities, this center of gravity shifts when we carry shoulder bags and use our arms and legs for reaching and balancing. Core stability enables us to coordinate these varied movements with grace and efficiency.

The Pilates Method Alliance (PMA) has recently articulated two additional Pilates principles, which could also be considered an extension of the principle of Centering: *whole body movements* and *balanced muscle development*.

Whole Body Movements

The Pilates system of movement is a holistic exercise program that emphasizes whole-body conditioning. This is one of the characteristics that make Pilates such a natural method for exploring fascial fitness concepts. Dynamic, whole-body movements and stretches are inherent in the Pilates repertoire, a departure from the single-muscle focus of traditional stretching and weight training. A fascial approach to exercise tends to focus on stretching and training long myofascial chains of muscles in movements that are more functional and intuitive, as an animal might move or stretch.

Balanced Muscle Development

Centering is not only about functionally coordinating the proximal and distal structures of the body. We can also think about it as achieving a functional balance of deep and superficial tissues (i.e., tissues proximal and distal to the joints). Later in this book, we discuss what happens when local (deep) stabilizers become inhibited and global (superficial) muscles become overactive or adopt a bracing strategy. Performing Pilates exercises under a watchful eye is an excellent way to identify and correct these patterns and we will show you how.

2. Concentration

Concentration is the *state of mind* we cultivate in a Pilates session. Joseph Pilates insisted that his exercises be performed purposefully (as opposed to, in his words, "just going through the motions"). To practice his method absent-mindedly, as just another set of callisthenic exercises, would mean missing out completely not only on the corrective nature of the system for the human structure, but also on its ability to revitalize one's entire sense of well-being.

Principles derived from both fascial and brain research support this idea. "Movement with Attention" is the first of Anat Baniel's nine essentials, and it states that, as the brain organizes the movement of the body, so does movement organize the structure of the brain. From a fascial perspective, we know that the fascia is home to ten times as many sensory nerve receptors as the muscles. When we move in a distracted or uninterested way, we restrict the communication of sensation to the central nervous system; this contributes to a habit of sensory dampening, which can lead to dysfunction and injury. In contrast, by paying attention to our movement, we are enhancing kinesthesia and proprioception, improving function over time and reducing the likelihood of injury.

We can think of the Pilates principle of Concentration as the principle that conveys the importance of our *state of mind* during exercise. There are several ways we can purposefully direct our state of mind during Pilates to unlock the full benefit of the exercises. Some suggestions from fascial and brain fitness include:

- **Awaring:** We can train our minds to be alert and aware (Baniel calls this awaring)—that is, we can generate awareness by noticing what is going on around us.
- **The learning switch:** We can learn to recognize whether the brain is in a learning state, or not. We only learn new things when we direct our attention towards learning— that is, when we turn the *learning switch* on. Baniel aims to activate the learning switch in her movement lessons, and so should we, as Pilates teachers and students.
- **Variety:** In order to remain alert and interested, the brain and the fascia require *variety*. Variation in activities can help you avoid getting stuck in rigid patterns of thinking, feeling, and being. When environments offer fresh and unexpected challenges, the mind and body stay awake and adaptable. The Pilates studio provides infinite ways to keep the mind engaged and the body pleasantly challenged. The Pilates apparatus enable us to work with different movement patterns in different planes of gravity. You should experiment also with movement *qualities* (e.g., tempo, micro-movements vs. fuller range, intensity, or "volume" of muscular contractions, focal points, etc.). Whatever you do, do not make the mistake of repeating the same routine or cues over and over again until you or your student begins to mentally "check out." To offer and receive the greatest benefits to mind and body, keep it fresh.
- **Enthusiasm:** Another Anat Baniel essential asks that we summon *enthusiasm* as a way of communicating to the brain that something we are working on is important. Like the previous examples, enthusiasm is a state of mind that puts the brain into a learning mode.

- **Pleasure:** One of the most effective ways to train the fascia, according to Tom Myers, is to follow the *pleasure principle*. In other words, moving in ways that feel good and natural, and noticing how you feel, is good for your brain *and* your fascia.

3. Breath

Joseph Pilates wrote that, before the full benefit of his method could be obtained, breathing must be corrected. Restoring the **Breath** is the *foundation* for Pilates. This process is a biomechanical, neurological, and even spiritual one.

As our constant companion, and our most immediate anchor to the present moment, the breath is a gateway to awareness. The simple act of focusing on the breath can have tremendous benefits for the autonomic nervous system, offering a shift out of our daily fight-or-flight, hustle-and-bustle state and into a state of relaxation. The brain-fortifying effects of meditation are well documented. If focusing on the breath for an hour a day were the only benefit of a regular Pilates practice, it would be life changing for many people.

But as it turns out, breathing is also a key component of core stability. We will discuss the biomechanics of breathing in a later chapter and we will also explore how to identify faulty breathing habits (and how to overcome them) with the help of the Pilates repertoire.

4. Control

Joseph Pilates originally called his exercise system *Contrology,* so named because he taught his students that if they practiced his exercises daily, complete control over all the movements of the body would result. **Control** was the *goal* of the Pilates system. This process of developing incredibly finely

tuned awareness and physical dexterity was what we today call *building kinesthesia*, kinesthetic intelligence (KI), or "waking up" areas of the body. For example, learning to roll through the spine, not treating it as one long board but as individual bones moving one at a time, demands a dynamic interplay between stability and mobility that is delicately coordinated by the nervous system.

If we consider control as the goal of Pilates, then we might consider Anat Baniel's eighth essential, "Imagination and Dreams," as a natural extension of this principle. "Imagination and Dreams" states that imagining new possibilities stimulates the neuronal connections in the brain and helps us overcome our present limitations. The Pilates principle of Control, which stems from Joe's radical idea that the average person could develop total mastery of the body (essentially "waking up" every muscle in the body), was visionary in his time, and still is today. What an inspiring possibility! This radically imaginative quality of Contrology's creator, the dream of new physical possibilities, is something that we as Pilates practitioners should strive to preserve. In doing so, we will be stimulating our minds and stretching ourselves to new levels that we may not have imagined for our practice.

5. Precision

Precision is the high *standard* asked of Pilates practitioners and teachers, and it is also the *prerequisite* for change.

This requirement for precision is the reason why the same Pilates exercise that is appropriate for a total beginner is just as likely to challenge a competitive athlete. Many people, including some athletes, have unwittingly adopted inefficient muscle activation strategies and have become good compensators in their activities of daily life and play. Through the requirement of precise stabilization and movement patterns, our individual weaknesses are revealed. This allows awareness of our usual patterns and helps us discover a more efficient approach.

Performing exercises correctly and with precision may require you to start all over, to become a beginner again. This can be unsettling at first, but to gloss over this principle is to proceed with a false sense of accomplishment, as overeager muscles may continue to dominate, masking the decline of the primary muscles better suited to the task. Whether athletes or desk jockeys, many of us have adopted some faulty compensatory patterns of movement, and these unfortunately take us only so far before we develop acute or chronic injuries. The reward of doing the precise work to correct these patterns is a deeply rooted strength that can sustain and enrich the body through a lifetime of physical activity.

To the Pilates principle of Precision, we can add the Anat Baniel essential, "Slow." The idea here is that you cannot make a change or master a new skill unless you slow down. Moving fast only grooves in patterns that are already automatic. Cueing a client to move slowly is a way to wake up the brain when it has fallen into a habitual mode of doing. Slowing down a great deal enhances perception and allows changes to be made.

Another Anat Baniel essential, "Subtlety," states that when we reduce the amount of force, we increase the brain's sensitivity and thus its ability to perceive differences (essential for the brain to learn and be successful). This essential supports the case for incorporating lower-load exercises into all training regimens, particularly those with a corrective aim. When we encounter chronically stiff or unstable patterns in our clients, we can conclude that these areas lack kinesthetic nuance. Bringing awareness of subtle differences through observation, touch cues, and rhetorical questions—such as "How does it feel when you lift here?"—can spark the brain's search for more-efficient movement choices.

6. Flow

Unlike the previous principle, where slow and precise movement is emphasized, **Flow** is the pinnacle expression, where we learn to bring the right amount of coordinated effort to the exercise, always recognizing and adjusting for jerky, bulging, heavy, or overly braced movements.

Psychologist Mihaly Csikszentmihalyi described Flow as a state of focused absorption in the activity in hand, in which the skill of the participant and the challenge of the activity are equally matched. The result is a sense of timeless, egoless engagement, not that different from what Anat Baniel describes as a state of total awareness in which the brain functions at its highest level.

Some Pilates teachers consider Flow as a reward to be enjoyed only once a student has mastered fundamental patterns. As the previous principle suggests, we cannot change our patterns when we move fast; we can only do what we already know how to do. For the beginning Pilates student, "flowing" for 60 minutes in a class setting is likely to direct their focus away from the kinesthetic nuances that are so important to, in Joe's words, "attaining physical and mental balance." If we are more focused on keeping up with others than on the subtle points of the exercise, then Pilates loses its depth and becomes just another group fitness class.

But at the same time that mastering foundations is important, flowing can also encourage sensory exploration and learning, especially when done to one's own rhythm. We suggest exploring basic movement patterns—that have also been learned slowly—in this way, and then moving on to compound movements. Executing choreography in sync with others makes a beautiful performance, but in a Pilates class, dance to your own inner rhythm and never sacrifice the other Pilates principles for this one.

We can add another dimension to our traditional understanding of Pilates Flow by considering the elastic nature of fascial tissue. We all are familiar with the idea that muscles contract and change length, pulling onto "passive" tendons, which cross the joints and generate movement. Fascia researchers have discovered another, highly efficient, mechanism of movement, referred to as the *catapult mechanism*, or *elastic recoil*. In this model, the muscles do not change length, but the fascial tissues store and release tension, like a spring; this is how kangaroos create their powerful jumps. Training with this mechanism in mind can improve resiliency and stamina in physical activities such as running. Fascial fitness specialists recommend incorporating bouncing movements, preparatory counter movements, and soft and flowing "ninja-like" hops into the movement repertoire. Whether through jumpboard work on the reformer, or creative adaptations of other Pilates repertoires, there is ample opportunity for training this elastic quality of the fascia within the Pilates context, and about which we will offer some ideas later in the book.

Other Tips from Fascial and Brain Research

Although the following ideas do not fit neatly within the six Pilates principles, they are useful tips for Pilates practitioners nonetheless:

- **Sustainability:** Fascia changes more slowly than muscle, and outside change may be hard to perceive right away. Have patience, because the cumulative effects will be felt and seen in the form of a stronger and more resilient fascial architecture.
- **Recovery and rest:** Pay attention and take regular, purposeful breaks to allow fascial tissue hydration.
- **Flexible goals:** Anat Baniel points out that we have as much to learn from failure as from success. Stay curious and encouraged, even when you cannot do an exercise.

The Functional Core

The Role of the Thoracopelvic Canister

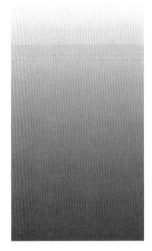

2

Joseph Pilates aptly named the core the "powerhouse" of the body. Throughout this book we will refer to the core, or the "powerhouse," as the *thoracopelvic canister* (TPC). The TPC consists of the thorax (thoracic spine and ribcage), the lumbar spine, and the pelvis. Together, this osseous framework, along with the soft tissue structures (muscles, fascia, and ligaments), forms an anatomical canister. Unlike an actual rigid canister, however, optimal function necessitates that the TPC also be flexible.

This chapter will discuss how core stability is developed, including which muscles are involved as well as the systems and strategies that are used to create optimal levels of stability for efficient movement. It will also look at the ramifications of a non-optimal TPC stabilization strategy for the development of common postural and movement dysfunction. The goal of this chapter is to leave you with the fundamental knowledge about how TPC (core) stabilization is achieved so that you:

- possess a working knowledge of how the TPC functions that is substantiated by a blend of the industry's best practices, available research, and clinical observations and anecdotes;
- have an understanding of how inefficient TPC stabilization strategies develop, and are able to identify the common signs of a dysfunctional strategy;
- have the tools and awareness to institute a corrective exercise strategy and progressive exercise program that helps you or your clients achieve lifelong health and fitness goals.

A highly integrated system is required for developing and maintaining optimal function of the TPC. How efficiently we are able to functionally control our TPC depends on the coordination of three key systems: the nervous system, the osseoligamentous system, and the myofascial system. These systems are seamlessly coordinated to provide the stability and control required to produce efficient posture and movement. While we will touch briefly upon each of the systems, the focus will be primarily on the myofascial system, since this system provides us with the access—a "way in," so to speak—required for developing, improving, and influencing the function of virtually every other system.

The Nervous System

The nervous system governs every function in the human body. It constantly monitors the information it receives from the proprioceptors located in the skin, muscles, fascia, ligaments, and joint capsules, as well as from the somatosensory system—the visual and vestibular systems—and uses this information to determine the most efficient strategy for stabilization and movement.

The nervous system is developed and maintained through the right amounts of diverse physical and intellectual stimulation. Child development perfectly exemplifies how neuroplastic we are in our early years; virtually every day it is possible to notice developing levels of motor control as well as increases in intellectual and emotional aptitude. These early months and years of development are crucial for forging the neural networks required for posture and movement throughout our lifetime. Crawling, for example, develops the TPC (core) and contralateral limb control that will ultimately be required for efficient upright posture and gait.

Improve Neural Connections
Unfortunately, because of our sedentary lifestyle, lack of diverse physical stimulation, and artificial types of exercise, our posture and movement patterns often begin to deteriorate. The great news is that because our nervous system retains neuroplastic qualities

throughout our lifetime, by incorporating the proper types and amounts of physical and intellectual challenges, we can improve at any age. Pilates then becomes an excellent medium through which we improve the neural connections—as well as develop some new ones—required for supporting a healthy and active lifestyle.

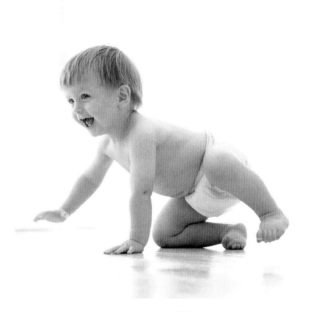

Figure 2.1: Crawling develops the TPC (core) and contralateral limb control.

Divisions of the Nervous System

The nervous system is the control system for our body; everything that happens within our body is driven by, and influences, the nervous system. It comprises two primary divisions (Figure 2.2): the central nervous system (CNS) and the peripheral nervous system (PNS). The brain and spinal cord make up the CNS, while the PNS is composed of the cranial and spinal nerves. The CNS processes and integrates the information provided by the PNS and sends out the appropriate commands required to elicit a specific activity or bodily function.

The PNS is further subdivided into the somatic and autonomic nervous systems. The somatic nervous system (SNS) controls the skeletal muscles, fascia, joints, and skin and is the region that controls our voluntary muscle activity. The autonomic nervous system (ANS) is responsible for our smooth muscle, cardiac muscles, and glands; essentially, it is involved in the bodily functions that keep us alive. Although it is largely under subconscious control, we can develop some control over our visceral, cardiac, and respiratory systems with conscious attention and through specific training. For example, through diaphragmatic breathing and getting into a relaxed mental state, we can consciously lower our heart and respiratory rates.

The ANS is further divided into the sympathetic (fight-or-flight) and parasympathetic (rest-and-digest) nervous systems. Because of our fast-paced lives, technology-driven overstimulation, lack of adequate rest, stimulant dependency (caffeine, medications, etc.), and daily responsibilities, many of us in this modern society live our lives in a sympathetic-dominant state. Being able to consciously lower our heart and respiratory rates through a proper breathing strategy is of huge benefit, as we can quickly move from a sympathetic-dominant state to a more parasympathetic one. The longer we are able to exist in a parasympathetic state, the more our bodies can efficiently carry out the functions required to thrive (digest, repair, detoxify, reduce inflammation, etc.) rather than just survive. This is an important component in developing overall health and longevity as well as in improving posture and movement.

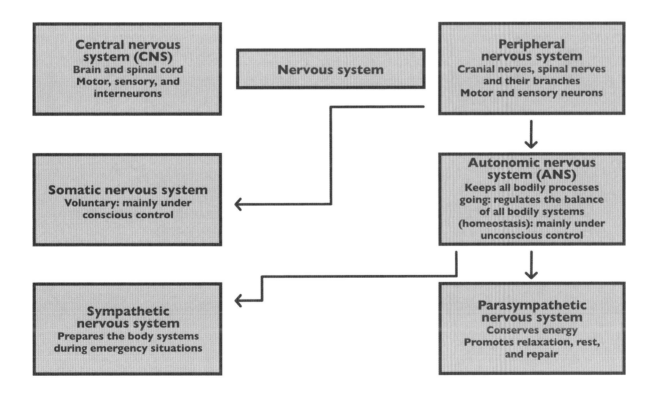

Figure 2.2: Central and peripheral nervous systems.

Exercise that creates fatigue, discomfort, and tissue breakdown—side effects associated with many of the high-intensity interval training (HIIT) methods—can easily perpetuate sympathetic nervous system dominance when performed at too great a frequency and duration, and without the proper rest or recuperation. This is a major cause of the chronic tightness and injuries we have seen in many of our clients and patients who regularly participate in these types of training program. HIIT methods are not necessarily bad if the individual can adequately handle the increased levels of stress; however, they are contraindicated for individuals with non-optimal posture and movement strategies as well as for those who are chronically fatigued or stressed.

Contrary to these HIIT types of approach, promoting a parasympathetic state is perhaps the biggest benefit of incorporating into a training program the Pilates principles of *breathing*, slowing movement down, and developing the *awareness* of conscious *control*. We have found great success in helping our clients and patients relieve chronic tension and discomfort, and even chronic inflammation associated with overuse, through regular incorporation of these principles.

Homunculus

The *homunculus* (pronounced ho-mun-cue-lous) is a pictorial representation of the motor and sensory regions of the brain. The homunculus man—or woman—represents the amount of space or attention that the brain devotes to different regions of the body.

As you can see in Figure 2.3, much of the focus of our brain's motor and sensory cortices is on our face, hands, and feet. This is one reason our children spend so much time looking, touching, tasting, listening, and grasping early in their development: they are providing information to the motor and sensory cortices and gaining valuable feedback required

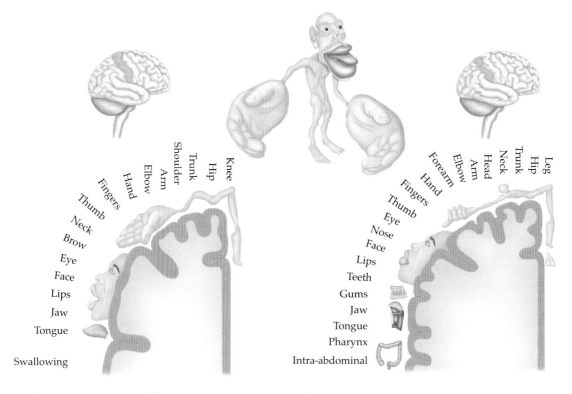

Figure 2.3: Pictorial representation of the motor and sensory regions of the brain.

for proper sensory and motor functions. In essence, they are developing their sense of proprioception—their awareness of position, location, orientation in space, and movement.

Where we have more awareness, the representation of these areas in the brain grows. Where we lack awareness, or have limited coordination and control, the representation of these areas in the brain is less. Throughout this book as we discuss improving efficiency and control in our movement habits, keep this image of homunculus in mind. Injury or trauma can cause the nervous system to have an impaired, or "smudged," representation of the injured area (for a great explanation of this, see Butler and Moseley 2013). Movement re-education—such as physical therapy, alignment-oriented yoga practices, and Pilates—aims to awaken awareness and control in areas that lack the *nuanced* strength which accompanies ideal function.

Note the child in Figure 2.4 stimulating both the motor and sensory divisions of her cerebral cortices. Tactile or kinesthetic feedback is an important component of re-educating and developing ideal postural and movement patterns. Performing Pilates exercises in bare feet, for example, is important for stimulating the peripheral receptors on the soles and relaying information back to the central nervous system about position, weight distribution, and direction of forces. The more we are able to provide a kinesthetically rich

environment, the more successful we can be at improving our patterns and, where required, develop more optimal habits. Remember the way we first learned as children and find as many ways as possible to incorporate some of these fundamentals into your Pilates practice.

It is important to note that every single activity we perform affects the nervous system. Every exercise then becomes an exercise in training or conditioning the nervous system. Thus the way you do an exercise is every bit as important as the exercise itself. The six Pilates principles described in Chapter 1 help us remember the state of mind behind the choreography. At whatever level you are practicing, from beginner to advanced, aim to embody these principles in your Pilates workout. This will forge neural pathways that spontaneously produce efficient and enjoyable movement patterns outside the Pilates studio.

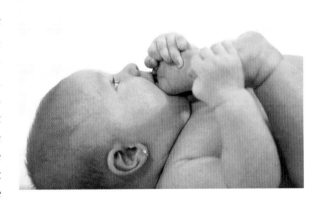

Figure 2.4: A child stimulating both the motor and sensory divisions of her cerebral cortices.

Be aware, Understand, and Concentrate
Every exercise is an opportunity to train or condition the nervous system. Check in with yourself before you exercise. Notice your breath, your mental state, your alignment, and how you are supporting your weight; take note especially of any tightness, aches, and/or pains. Ask yourself, "How will the exercise I am about to perform and the manner in which I am performing it influence the nervous system?" In this way, awareness, understanding, and concentration can be powerful tools for our Pilates practice, quietly transforming body, mind, and spirit as we move.

The Osseoligamentous System

The *osseous* component of the TPC refers to the bones that form the structural framework of our body. The bones that comprise the TPC or proximal core (Figure 2.5) include the following:

• thorax—thoracic spine, ribs, and sternum

• lumbar spine

• pelvis

Our bony architecture serves three important functions:

1. It acts as a stacked frame to increase our overall vertical height, thereby extending our capacity for locomotion, reach, and vision.

2. It enables us to use bones as levers, providing the ability to develop strength as well as to reach and rotate to achieve an almost infinite number of angles and positions.

3. It provides fixed attachment points so that contraction of the myofascial system is coordinated and organized in producing efficient posture and movement.

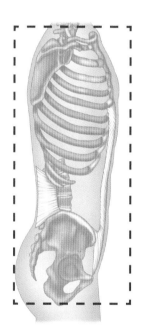

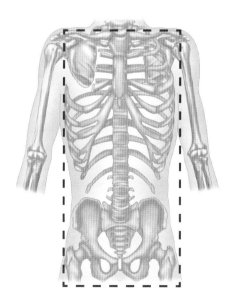

Figure 2.5: The thoracopelvic canister (TPC).

One additional function relating to posture and movement is that the periosteum—the fibrous sheath surrounding the bones—contains sensory receptors. In essence, our bones also serve a proprioceptive function.

The unique architecture of the alternating lordotic (cervical and lumbar) and kyphotic (thoracic) curvatures (Figure 2.6) enables the spine to work as a functional shock absorber for handling compressive forces coming either from above (gravity and external loading) or from below (the transfer of forces up through the body from contact of the foot with the ground). (The ability to dissipate shock would be greatly diminished if the spine were a completely straight rod.) Increases or decreases in these spinal curvatures then create biomechanical challenges that often become causes of stress to the soft tissue structures and lead to degenerative joint changes within the body. We will cover some of these challenges in a later section.

The trunk and spine (axial skeleton) is an attachment point for the head, as well as for the upper and lower extremities (appendicular skeleton). The lower extremities are attached to the TPC via the femoroacetabular (hip) joints, while the only bony attachment of the upper extremities to the axial skeleton is via the sternoclavicular articulations. Through the myofascial chains, the extremities contribute to stabilization, so the contribution from the extremities cannot be left out of a discussion on core function. We explore this concept further in the myofascial and exercise sections.

Additionally, the osseous structures of the TPC surround and protect the spinal cord and most of the body's vital organs that are located within the thorax, abdomen, and pelvis. As we will discover in the myofascial section, the TPC furnishes the structural support that provides suspension of the abdominal organs.

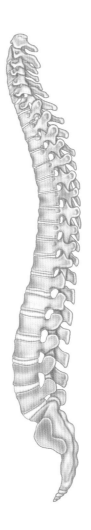

Figure 2.6: The spinal curvatures—cervical lordosis, thoracic kyphosis, and lumbar lordosis.

The ligamentous system supports and provides a level of stability to our joints. Ligaments connect two articulating (adjoining) bones and fascially blend with the joint capsule, which, in addition to providing fascial connections to the surrounding muscles, offers stability and varying degrees of mobility based on the joint's unique structure and function. The majority of joints in our trunk, spine, pelvis, and extremities, as well as in the osseous structures of the TPC, are synovial—that is, they contain a joint capsule, synovial fluid, and two articulating cartilage-covered bones (Figure 2.7).

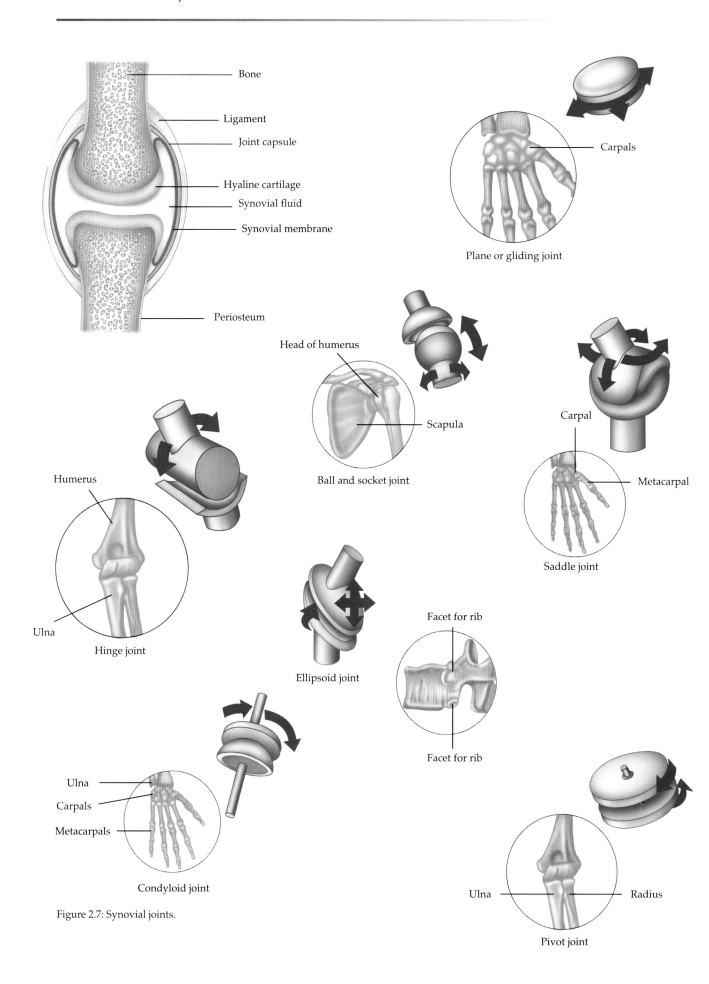

Figure 2.7: Synovial joints.

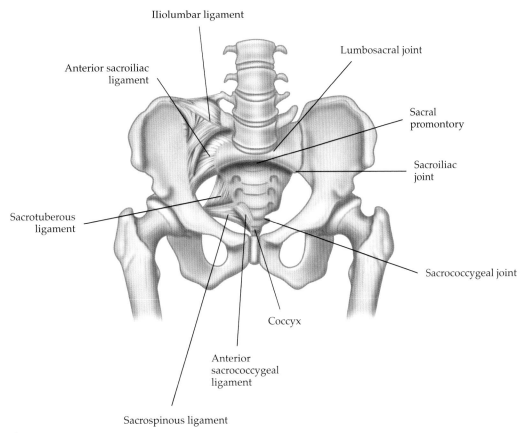

Iliolumbar ligament

Anterior sacroiliac ligament

Lumbosacral joint

Sacral promontory

Sacroiliac joint

Sacrotuberous ligament

Sacrococcygeal joint

Coccyx

Anterior sacrococcygeal ligament

Sacrospinous ligament

Figure 2.8: The sacroiliac joint.

While it has long been known that ligaments and joint capsules are densely innervated by sensory neurons (proprioceptors), it is now recognized that much of our posture control is modulated by means of ligaments. Muscles contract and pull on their fascial attachments to ligaments in order to provide joint stability. Although they were once thought of as merely passive restraints to joint motion, recent evidence suggests that many biological tissues, including the ligaments and surrounding fibrous connective tissue, have less organized but similar properties. They contain contractile elements that enable them to respond in a mechanically stiffening or stabilizing manner (Schleip et al. 2012). In other words, all the tissues surrounding a joint are as important for transmitting information back to the nervous system as they are for providing joint stability.

The bones' various shapes and the types of joints they form also determine how inherently stable a region of the body will be. Based on each bone's unique architecture, the propensity towards stability of certain joint articulations is greater, while others are better designed for mobility. The sacroiliac joints (SIJs) of the pelvis, for example, are considered to have a greater level of inherent stability, or *form closure*—a term coined by Andry Vleeming and Chris Snijders (Lee 2011). The rather unique design of the SIJs (Figure 2.8) provides the stability needed for the transference of force from the extremities up through the trunk and spine, and from the trunk and spine down into the extremities.

The articulating surfaces of the sacrum and pelvis have irregular cartilage surfaces that "grip" onto each other as they join together.

The arrowhead-shaped sacrum is functionally wedged between the two innominate bones and held together by strong, dense ligaments. These unique arrangements create a significant degree of inherent stability, or form closure, of the sacroiliac joints. We will discuss how the myofascial system contributes to the stability (force closure) of the sacroiliac joint in the next section.

The glenohumeral joint (Figure 2.9), by contrast, consists of a relatively large humeral head that articulates with the glenoid fossa of the scapula. This relationship allows significant range of motion through the joint, but the joint lacks the inherent stability of the sacroiliac joint. Therefore, the glenohumeral joint relies significantly upon the myofascial system to provide the control needed to maintain joint stability through functional activities.

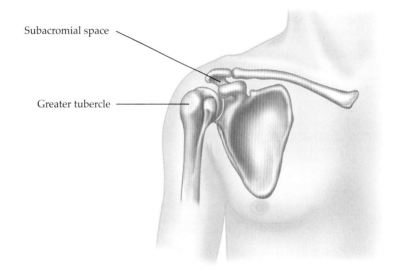

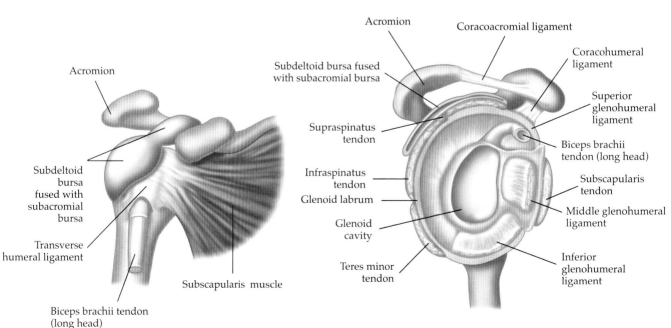

Figure 2.9: The glenohumeral joint. Notice the relatively larger humeral head as it articulates with the smaller glenoid fossa of the scapula. This arrangement requires control provided by the joint capsule and the investing rotator cuff muscles.

Regardless of the amount of form closure a joint possesses, the ligaments and shape of the joint are not enough to provide the support required for upright posture and movement. Thus all joints depend on the myofascial system to support, accelerate, and/or decelerate the body without creating unwanted stresses to the joint and soft tissue structures.

The Myofascial (Muscle + Fascial) System

As described in Chapter 1, fascia is a "web"—a connective tissue that envelops, suspends, supports, and invests all of the structures of the body. The *myofascial system* refers to the interwoven and inseparable nature of the muscles and the fascia. Together, the myofascial system creates stability (integrity) in the body through tensile forces, which can be either compressive or decompressive in nature.

Tensegrity (tension + integrity) is an architectural model developed by Buckminster Fuller, which describes a continuous tension-generating system in which tensile cords connect to non-continuous rigid levers. This design provides the benefit of being "light," while also having an inherent stability *and* adaptability. The fascial system of the human body has been called the *organ of stability* and *mechano-regulation* (Myers 2011, citing Varela and Frenk), meaning that its job is to do just that—provide stability and maintain it by adapting to whatever mechanical forces it encounters.

Before the tensegrity model was applied to the human body, we tended to think of the body's stability as simply a function of compressive forces (i.e., gravity and ground reaction force), like the stacked bricks in a building.

Today, we understand that the body develops its own internal cohesion, responding to constantly variable demands on its stability through an intricate fascial tensegrity. In the application of the tensegrity concept to our body, the myofascial system functions as the tension-generators while our bones form a

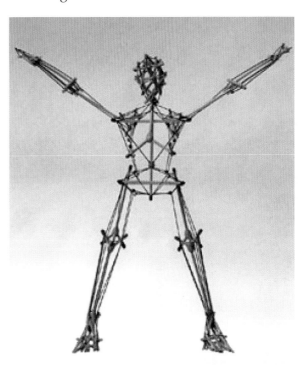

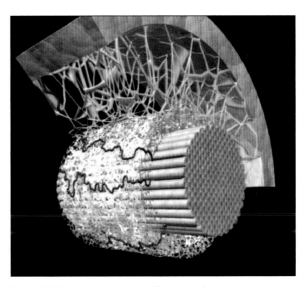

Figure 2.10: A tensegrity model (top image) and a conceptualization in the human body (bottom image). The bottom image is reproduced with the kind permission of Dr. J.C. Guimberteau and Endovivo Productions.

non-continuous, interconnected, rigid lever system (Figure 2.10). We will examine both the compressive and decompressive roles of the myofascial system in this chapter.

Really, It Is the Neuro-Myo-Fascial System
It has been said that muscles are a window to the brain (Butler et al. 2013). Truly, our thoughts, emotions, and beliefs are reflected in our posture and movement patterns and the mechanical tensions associated with them. (And vice versa, by the way. Check out Amy Cuddy's excellent TED Talk on the subject.) Once again, we return to the wisdom of the Pilates principles, which emphasize how the *state of mind* when we exercise is an integral part of the development of optimal postural and movement patterns.

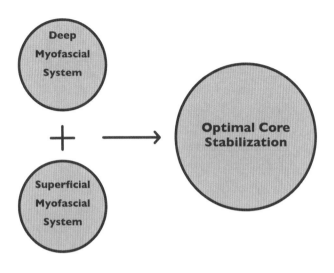

Figure 2.11: When there is balance between the deep and superficial myofascial systems, optimal core stabilization is achieved.

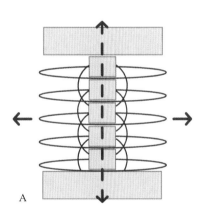

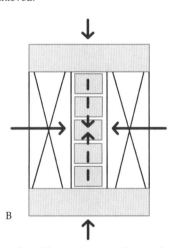

Figure 2.12: (a) The muscles of the DMS are arranged circumferentially around, and/or are segmentally attached directly to, the bones of the TPC; (b) the muscles of the SMS are vertically oriented or crossed (X shape) along the TPC.

The deep and superficial myofascial systems, coordinated by the nervous system, work synergistically to support the development of optimal TPC (core) stabilization and movement patterns. Incorporation of the Pilates principles is one of the best ways to ensure development of balance between these two systems.

The muscles of the deep myofascial system (DMS) tend to be arranged circumferentially around, and/or are segmentally attached directly to, the bones of the TPC (Figure 2.12(a)). In contrast, the muscles of the superficial myofascial system (SMS) tend to be vertically oriented or crossed (X shape) along the TPC (Figure 2.12(b)). The transversus abdominis, part of the DMS, is a circumferentially oriented muscle that fascially blends into the thoracolumbar fascia and attaches to each level of the lumbar spine, the lower aspect of the ribcage, and the upper rim of the pelvis.

In contrast, the abdominal obliques, part of the SMS, lie more superficially attaching from the external aspect of the ribcage to the pelvis. While these muscles have a significant impact upon function of the TPC, they do not have the same level of control over each vertebral segment as compared with the deep system. However, both systems contribute to efficient stabilization and optimal movement, as we will discuss.

Several individuals, including Richardson and colleagues, Jull, and Janda, have categorized muscles based on their function (Chaitow et al. 2014) and location (Lee 2011). Our categorization synthesizes their work and considers the individualized function of muscles as supported by the research. For simplicity, we will refer to the muscles of the TPC (core) in terms of the deep and superficial myofascial systems.

The distinction between whether a muscle is part of the deep myofascial system or the superficial myofascial system is determined by five primary characteristics: the muscle's location, size, proprioceptive density, functional role, and response to dysfunction (Table 2.1). We will look first at the characteristics and specific muscles that comprise the deep myofascial system.

Characteristics	Deep Myofascial System	Superficial Myofascial System
Location	• deep to intermediate • near axis of rotation	• intermediate to superficial • further from axis of rotation
Size	• small-to-medium fiber size • primarily type I or IIa oxidative muscle fibers	• medium-to-large fiber size • primarily type IIa or IIb glycolytic muscle fibers
Proprioception	• dense • feed forward: anticipatory activation	• relatively sparse • feed back: responsive activation
Functional role	• low-level activity • low threshold level to recruitment • segmental stabilization • fine motor and postural control • non-specific directional control	• high-level activity • high threshold level to recruitment • gross stabilization • large movement • shock absorption • direction-specific activity
Response to dysfunction	• inhibition, including recruitment delays, decreased force production, decreased endurance • atrophy	• over-activation • lower threshold to firing • over-recruitment, with decreased ability to relax when not required • hypertonicity

Table 2.1: Comparison of the characteristics of the deep and superficial myofascial systems.

Deep Myofascial System

As the name implies, the deep myofascial system consists of the muscles that lie deep to the superficial muscles and contain the deep-to-intermediate layers of musculature. These muscles tend to be smaller and intersegmental, meaning they directly connect one or two joint segments in the spine and one bone to another in the periphery of the body. They lie close to the axis of rotation (theoretical center-point where the joint rotates), which provides them with the ability to exert control and make specific adjustments to the joints.

The muscles that lie close to the joint, in this case the multifidi in Figure 2.13, fascially blend with the ligaments and joint capsules and have a better ability to monitor and control small movements of the joint. This provides a more specific level of joint control than that of the superficial (erector spinae) muscles, which tend to be located further from the axis of rotation and generally cross more than one joint segment.

The muscles of the deep system primarily comprise tonic, or type I, oxidative fibers, meaning they use oxygen for energy. This constitution allows the deep muscles to maintain constant activity, whereas muscles that depend primarily on glycogen for energy—like the muscles of the superficial system—are quick to fatigue. Endurance is a critical feature of the deep muscles, as they need to maintain constant monitoring and control of the joints. Even at rest, there is generally a low level of activity in these muscles. We want these deeper muscles, which tend to be our joint stabilizers, to always exert some level of control and not to be simply contracting and relaxing (turning on and off), which commonly occurs after an injury.

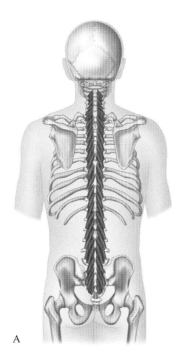
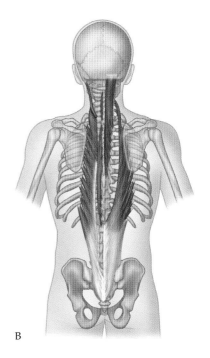

A   B

Figure 2.13: The deep myofascial system. Note how the deeper muscles of the spine—here the multifidi (a.)—attach directly to each one or two levels of the spine, whereas the superficial erector spinae (b.) muscles span many more levels.

Two additional benefits of these deeper muscles are that they tend to have non-specific and feed-forward activity. *Non-specificity* refers to their ability to contract regardless of the motion of the trunk and spine, and unlike the superficial muscles their activation is not position or activity dependent. In other words, there is always some level of activity in these muscles regardless of body position or direction of movement. These muscles are also *feed-forward* muscles, meaning they contract milliseconds before the prime movers (which tend to be our superficial muscles); this is an important function that allows joint stabilization prior to movement.

The feed-forward aspect appears to be present in many of the deeper muscles, including the transversus abdominis, pelvic floor, diaphragm, and multifidi. This important function allows joint stabilization prior to creating actual movement. For example, before lifting your chest for the Hundred or any of the exercises in the Pilates Ab Series, you want your deep myofascial system to activate and stabilize your core (TPC). If the deep stabilizers of the spine and pelvis fail to pre-activate and stabilize your joints, the pull of the more superficial rectus abdominis and abdominal obliques, and/or the movement of the extremities, would disrupt the alignment of your trunk, spine, and pelvis, creating a compensated movement pattern and potential injuries. This pre-activation of the deep core is the first step to facilitating TPC (core) stability and control in all Pilates exercises, from Leg Circles and Side Kick series to more difficult movement patterns such as the Pilates Teaser (Figure 2.14).

We want the muscles of the deep myofascial system to always exert some level of control and not simply be turning on and off at random times, which typically happens when there is injury, trauma, or stress to the system. We will discuss this further in a later chapter. During palpation of the abdominal wall, on either yourself or your client, you should note a pre-activation of the deep abdominal wall that occurs independently of the superficial abdominal muscles (Figure 2.15). This activation should not cause excessive tone in the superficial muscles and/or cause a change in the neutral alignment of the TPC.

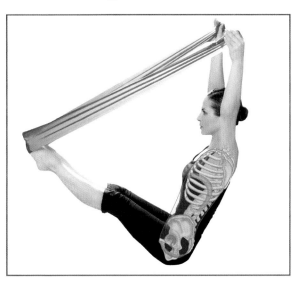

Figure 2.14: The Pilates Teaser. Prior to lifting of the arms and legs, the deep myofascial system is activated to stabilize the TPC.

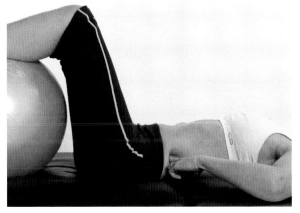

Figure 2.15: Individual pre-activating her deep myofascial system.

Muscles of the deep myofascial system include, but are not limited to, the transversus abdominis, psoas, diaphragm, pelvic floor, multifidi, quadratus lumborum, rotatores, interspinalis, intertransversarii, levator costarum, and intercostalis (Table 2.2). Note in Figure 2.16 how the muscles and investing fascia of the deep myofascial system create a myofascial girdle around the thorax, spine, and pelvis. This provides the ability to control segmental stability and contribute to the production of smooth and efficient movement.

It may seem that certain muscles listed in the deep myofascial system—the transversus abdominis and psoas, for example—are quite large muscles; and indeed they are, if you consider their sheer size and expansiveness. However, because each has specific fascial attachments to the bones and ligaments of the spine, thorax, and pelvis, in addition to fascial attachments to a multitude of other deep muscles, they can exert segmental control of the spine, thorax, and pelvis, thereby functioning just as though they were physically attached between one joint segment and the next.

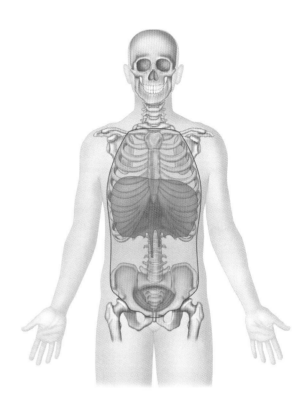

Figure 2.16: The myofascial girdle around the thorax, spine, and pelvis created by the muscles and investing fascia of the deep myofascial system.

Deep Myofascial System	Superficial Myofascial System
Diaphragm	Anterior and posterior oblique chains
Transversus abdominis	Flexor and extensor chains
Pelvic floor	Lateral chain
Psoas	Deep longitudinal chain
Multifidi	
Rotatores	
Interspinalis	
Intertransversarii	
External/internal intercostalis	
Levator costarum	

Table 2.2: Examples of the muscles of the deep and superficial myofascial systems of the core.

Note: Certain muscles, such as the quadratus lumborum, psoas, multifidi, and erector spinae, contain characteristics that could technically place them in either category. The deeper fibers of these muscles have divisions that share characteristics with the deep myofascial system, while the superficial fibers share traits that are characteristic of the superficial myofascial system. For simplicity, we will consider muscles as belonging to one group or the other.

The Role of the Fascial Envelope in TPC Stability

The inherent efficiency of the body operating as a tensegrity model is apparent when we consider how core stability is generated through the fascial envelope. You can envision this mechanism as a balloon (representing a muscle or group of muscles) being surrounded by a piece of elastic tubing (the fascia). When the balloon is only semi-inflated, there is relatively little tension being placed on the elastic tubing; this is an example of a relaxed muscle inside its fascial envelope. However, as the balloon expands (the muscle contracts) against the elastic tubing (the fascial envelope), the elastic tubing is pulled taut.

In our body, consider the multifidi as the balloon and the thoracolumbar fascia that surrounds them as the elastic tubing. As the transversus abdominis (which fascially connects into the thoracolumbar fascia) contracts and tensions the thoracolumbar fascia, the contraction of the multifidi swells or pushes out into the fascial envelope (formed by the thoracolumbar fascia), thereby stabilizing the vertebral segment underneath.

One interesting aspect of this stabilization model is that research into the preferential activation of these single-joint, intersegmental stabilizer muscles—such as the multifidi, transversus abdominis, and pelvic floor—has demonstrated that activating them develops the appropriate levels of tension required to stabilize the joints (Richardson et al. 2004). It is the uncontrolled shear and rotational stresses that tend to wear out our joint cartilage while placing high levels of potentially damaging stress upon soft tissue structures, such as the intervertebral discs of the spine. It is important for physical trainers to recognize that the intersegmental joint control (control of one vertebral segment on an adjoining vertebral segment) necessary in order to resist these forces requires the generation of only a relatively small amount of muscle contraction by the deep myofascial system.

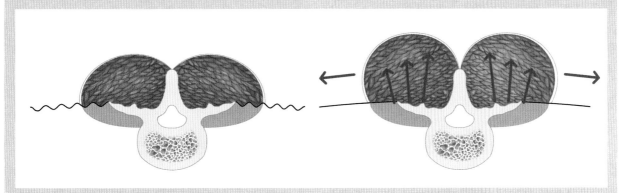

Figure 2.17. Schematic representation of tensegrity at work in the spine. When the transversus abdominis and multifidi are relaxed, the vertebra is able to move in relationship to its neighbor. When contraction of the transversus abdominis tensions the thoracolumbar fascia so that it is pulled taut over the muscle, the contraction of the multifidi against the surrounding thoracolumbar fascia stiffens the vertebral segment, thereby stabilizing it against movement.

Superficial Myofascial System

The superficial myofascial system consists of the intermediate-to-superficial layers of muscles. These are the larger muscles—those that tend to span two or more joint segments and are located further from the axis of rotation. These muscles are primarily composed of type II glycolytic fibers—that is, they use glycogen for energy, which allows them to contract fast and hard. However, because they use glycogen for energy, they tend to fatigue quickly. While the superficial muscles also contain proprioceptors, they typically have a lower percentage than the deeper muscles, so they are not as sensitive to subtle changes in joint motion as the deeper muscles. It generally takes larger perturbations or disruptions to joint motion or body position to enable the superficial muscles to detect this motion and relay signals back to the central nervous system, which is not an efficient system of control. If inhibition of the DMS persists following an initial trauma, the low sensitivity (and resulting over-activity) of the SMS becomes a common cause of recurring injury even after the muscle and soft tissues of the joint have adequately healed.

Muscles of the superficial myofascial system include, but are not limited to, the anterior and posterior oblique chains, flexor and extensor chains, lateral chain, deep longitudinal chain (Table 2.2). The superficial muscles function to create general, or gross, stabilization and movement. This means that because they are located relatively far from the axis or center of rotation, they cannot specifically control or move the joint like the deeper muscles.

Additionally, their activity is direction specific, meaning they are only turned on by a specific direction of movement. By virtue of these characteristics, their action on the joints is usually compressive and non-specific; thus they tend to pull the joint out of alignment if not balanced by the deeper myofascial system.

Consider the Side Sit-Up on the Reformer Short Box (Figure 2.18). As the individual lowers herself into a left side-bend, her right external oblique is eccentrically contracting (lengthening) to control her motion. The left external oblique (superficial myofascial system) is relatively quiet during this pattern, as it does not need to activate to assist this motion. However, the transversus abdominis (TVA) (as part of the deep myofascial system) will be constantly activated beneath both sets of obliques, as it must control the trunk, spine, and pelvis throughout all ranges of the exercise. If the TVA is unable to perform this stabilizing function, the resulting compression and shearing forces on the intervertebral discs can cause serious injury to the spine.

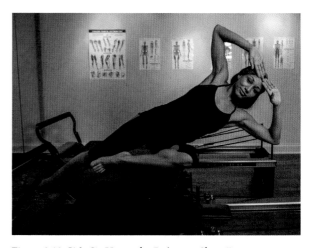

Figure 2.18: Side Sit-Up on the Reformer Short Box.

Myofascial Chains

While muscles tend to be taught as discrete entities with separate and individual functions, when you are aiming to improve posture and/or movement they should also be understood in an expanded context. When viewed in a broader context, all muscles are fascially connected to other muscles, forming longer functional myofascial units (Figure 2.19). These connected myofascial units have been described using a variety of terms, including *myofascial slings* by Tittel, *muscle chains* by Kabat, Struyf-Dens, Busquet and others (Schleip et al. 2012), and simply *fascial chains* (Paoletti 2006). The connecting nature of the fascial matrix has also been instrumental in the development of the "mechanical link in osteopathy" by Chauffor (Schleip et al. 2012) and "anatomy trains" by Myers (2014). Several of the myofascial lines as described by Myers are represented in Table 2.3, overleaf.

The myofascial chains link regions of the body together and function to increase the amplitude of stabilization, acceleration, or deceleration of the body. Given the intricate weaving of the fascial system, there are theoretically innumerable muscular chains working to stabilize and move the body at any given moment.

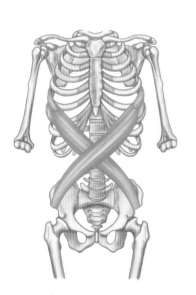 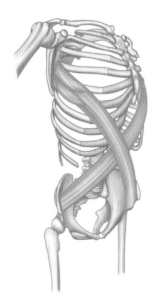 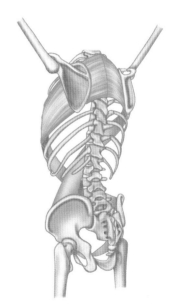

Figure 2.19: An example of the continuity of the myofascial lines or chains.

Anatomy Train	Myofascial Components	
Anterior spiral line	splenius capitis (contralateral), rhomboids, serratus anterior, external oblique abdominal, abdominal fascia, internal oblique abdominal (contralateral), adductor complex (contralateral)	
Posterior spiral line	latissimus dorsi (contralateral), thoracolumbar fascia, gluteus maximus and tensor fasciae latae, iliotibial band, peroneus longus	
Superficial back line	plantar fascia, short toe flexors, gastrocnemius, hamstring complex, erector spinae, occipital fascia	
Superficial front line	sternocleidomastoid, sternalis, rectus abdominis, quadriceps, tibialis anterior, extensor digitorum	
Lateral line	splenius capitis/cervicis–sternocleidomastoid/scalenes, external intercostals–internal intercostals, external abdominal obliques–internal abdominal obliques, gluteus maximus–tensor fasciae latae, gluteus medius and contralateral quadratus lumborum, extensor digitorum longus/peroneus tertius–tibialis anterior	

Table 2.3: Several of the myofascial lines as described by Myers.

Notes:

1. All muscles are referenced to the same side of the body unless the chain crosses the midline, in which case they are indicated as contralateral (e.g., anterior and posterior oblique chains).

2. Muscles of the lateral chain are paired by the nature of how they criss-cross each other; these are separated by a dash (–).

3. Many muscles, such as the latissimus dorsi, erector spinae, and peroneus longus, function as part of multiple chains.

4. Certain chains, such as the flexor and extensor, the lateral, and the arm flexor and extensor chains, include the same muscles bilaterally.

Whereas the muscles of the deep myofascial system are more responsible for specific joint control, the superficial myofascial chains are required for accelerating and decelerating the body as well as for higher levels of stabilization. These myofascial chains enable us to create the necessary movements of life—that is, the fundamental movement patterns that include squatting, lunging, pushing, pulling, bending, rotating, and walking. Every movement in life is, in essence, composed of one or more combinations of these fundamental patterns. For example, bending over to pick up your child and lifting them overhead requires a combination of the squatting or bending pattern to get down to the level of your child, a pulling pattern to lift them from the ground in towards your center of gravity, and a pushing pattern to lift them up overhead.

The fundamental movement patterns can be trained in isolation and then in combination by incorporating a variety of Pilates patterns into your repertoire. Analyzing a particular movement pattern where a client struggles or experiences pain allows us to break that movement down into its fundamental components and effectively train improved control. This element of the Pilates system enables virtually anyone to enhance their performance, whether their goal is to play with their children, participate in their sport, or move more efficiently so that they experience less chronic tightness and pain.

The Fascial System

Although fascia was once considered simply a white fibrous connective tissue, recent exploration into the fascial system brings an entirely new perspective to this dynamic structure. While fascia is connected to virtually every structure in our body down to the cellular level, it serves several important functions in terms of developing a core stabilization strategy.

1. Fascia joins all our connective tissue into one functional unit and plays an important role in maintaining integrity within the entire body. On a more superficial level, fascia connects tendon to ligament, ligament to joint capsule on one side of a joint, and joint capsule to another corresponding ligament and musculotendinous junction on the opposing side of the joint. This provides the continuous flexibility and stability required to support and stabilize the joints in both posture and movement.

2. Another important role of this fascial network is that it suspends both our visceral system (organs) and the structure of our entire body. While the bones provide the architectural framework and anchor points, it is the fascial system that provides the suspensory support required for upright posture and movement as well as for optimal organ function.

On intermediate and deeper levels, fascia surrounds and protects our blood vessels, lymph vessels, and nerves. Periosteum—a specialized layer of fascia surrounding our bones—connects into the muscular fascia and also functions in the roles of protection and proprioception.

3. Fascia contains structures known as *myofibroblasts*—a contractile variant of fibroblasts (Schleip et al. 2012). Previously it was thought that myofibroblasts' primary role was in wound healing and the development of pathological conditions such as Dupuytren's contracture or frozen shoulder (Schleip et al. 2012). However, myofibroblasts have been shown to be present in various samples of fascial tissue—including the thoracolumbar (lumbodorsal) fascia, iliotibial band, and plantar fascia—which suggests their ubiquity in all fascia (Schleip et al. 2102). The myofibroblasts provide fascia with the ability to contribute to stability, dissipate forces along different lines of fascia, and maintain a level of flexibility and adaptability within the entire musculoskeletal–fascial system.

4. Proprioception—the conscious and subconscious perception of our body in space and in movement—is an important component of developing an efficient postural and movement strategy. Fascia contains specialized mechanoreceptors that make it an extension of the nervous system in the control of posture and movement (Schleip et al. 2012). These mechanoreceptors respond to mechanical pressure (such as pressure, tension, and stretching) and—along with information received from the skin, eyes, and vestibular system—supply the nervous system with the information it requires to develop conscious and subconscious control of posture and movement.

All of the factors above, attributable to the fascial system, allow the various body systems (cardiovascular, pulmonary, gastrointestinal, urogenital, osseoligamentous, and muscular) to operate as one functional unit. Thus overall body function is driven by the fascial system, and dysfunction will also be reflected in this system (Paoletti 2006).

Let's consider the deep longitudinal myofascial chain of the anterior tibialis, peroneus longus, long head of the biceps femoris, sacrotuberous ligaments, sacroiliac joint ligaments, thoracolumbar fascia, and contralateral erector spinae during the foot contact phase of the gait cycle. Keep in mind that while we move primarily in a forward or sagittal plane of motion during gait, it is really the neuro-myofascial control of the multiple rotating segments within the kinetic chain that enables us to transfer these rotational forces into the linear motion of walking.

As the heel contacts the ground, concentric contraction of the anterior tibialis (along with the advancement of the forward leg) eccentrically stretches the posterior components of the deep longitudinal chain. As a result, the tension created in the peroneus longus produces tension in its fascial connection at the long head of the biceps femoris, which in turn tensions its fascial connection to the sacrotuberous ligament (Figure 2.20).

This causes tension in the deep contralateral erector spinae, myofascially attached to the sacroiliac joint through the thoracolumbar fascia, which stabilizes the pelvis and spine as the body moves forward. The action of the erector spinae also helps control or dampen some of the rotary forces that are occurring through the spine by virtue of the leg and

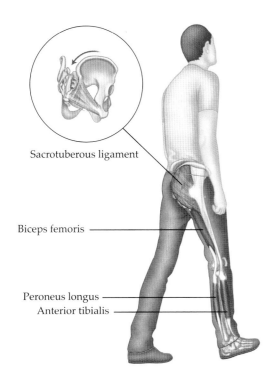

Sacrotuberous ligament

Biceps femoris

Peroneus longus
Anterior tibialis

Figure 2.20: The linear motion of walking: eccentric stretching of the posterior components of the deep longitudinal chain; tensioning of the biceps femoris' fascial connection to the sacrotuberous ligament.

pelvis moving forward on one side while the trunk is rotating in the opposite direction.

These collective actions pull the sacrotuberous ligament, sacroiliac ligaments, and investing fascia taut, and this serves to lock the sacroiliac joint so that it is stable and provides the support we need as we move into single-leg stance. This is an ingenious design in that it creates stability, control of rotational forces, and transmission of forces across the body, resulting in smooth and coordinated gait.

How can Pilates improve the integrative function of the fascial system? Visualize this myofascial chain when performing Going Up Front on the Chair (Figure 2.21), or the lunge pattern in the Core Align Lunge with Twist (Figure 2.22). In both cases, the foot, leg, and pelvis must remain stable and aligned. Working slowly, with a focus on precision, will reveal where control is lacking along the myofascial

chain. By correcting the alignment of the foot, ankle, knee, and hips, while encouraging elongation of the deep core and releasing gripping patterns in the superficial myofascial system, you can begin to develop a more efficient and sustainable movement pattern.

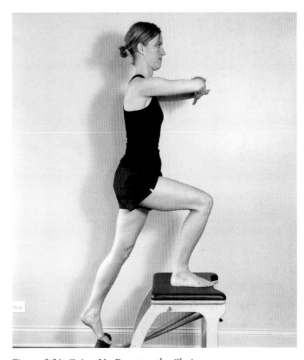

Figure 2.21: Going Up Front on the Chair.

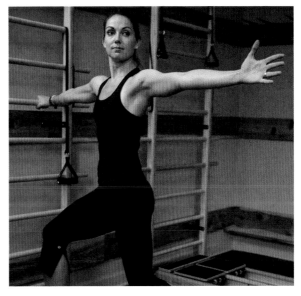

Figure 2.22: Core Align Lunge with Twist.

Fascial Tensegrity in Stabilization

Another example of how we use tensegrity in stabilizing the pelvis and ultimately our spine occurs during the gait cycle. As you are walking and come into the mid-stance phase of the gait cycle (the point at which your foot is flat on the ground and you are supported on one leg), there is a tremendous requirement to stabilize your pelvis and bodyweight over your stance leg while also controlling the advancement or forward momentum of your body. The stability required to assist your core in this task is provided by contraction of the gluteus maximus and tensor fasciae latae (TFL), which creates tension in the iliotibial band (ITB), pulling it taut against the lateral thigh. The vastus lateralis, sitting just beneath the ITB, then contracts to straighten the knee and pushes out against the now-taut ITB (Figure 2.23). This sequence of events transforms the lower extremity into a solid lever that can effectively support us in single-leg stance.

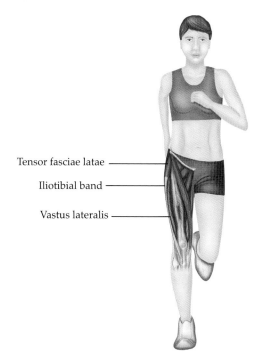

Tensor fasciae latae

Iliotibial band

Vastus lateralis

Figure 2.23: Stabilizing the pelvis during the gait cycle: the ITB is pulled against the lateral thigh, and then the vastus lateralis contracts to straighten the knee.

Fascial Tensegrity in Controlling Rotation

Rotation is a necessary component of efficient gait and movement. Fascial tensegrity plays an integral role in producing and controlling rotary forces across the body. The loss of efficient rotary control is a leading cause of non-contact injuries (i.e., injuries in which there is no direct trauma to the body) as well as of decreased efficiency in control of posture and movement.

The oblique chains fascially connect the contralateral upper and lower extremities across the trunk; this enables these chains to "wind up" and eccentrically load prior to releasing the stored elastic tension (and concentric contraction) to create acceleration (Figure 2.24). This ability to use the tension created within the myofascial system enables us to use less overall effort when performing activities such as walking and to maximize these myofascial forces when we are accelerating either our body (in running and sprinting, for example) or an object (such as throwing a ball or swinging a golf club).

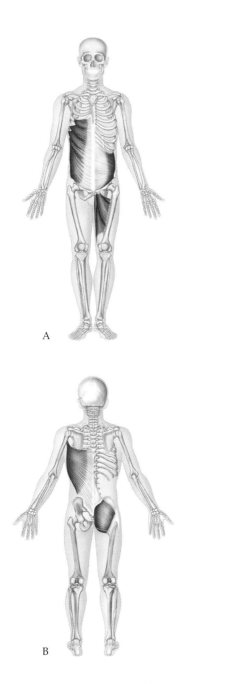

A

B

Figure 2.24: The anterior (a) and posterior (b) oblique chains make activities such as walking and running smooth and coordinated. Using the elastic energy that is stored up by the active and passive tensioning of the adjoining myofascial structures, we are able to produce and control rotary forces through our body, making movement more efficient while reducing potentially damaging stresses on our joints and soft tissue.

Pilates exercises such as Saw, Snake-Twist, Single-Arm Push-Ups, and Criss-Cross (Figure 2.25) are examples of Pilates movements that incorporate specific training of the oblique chains.

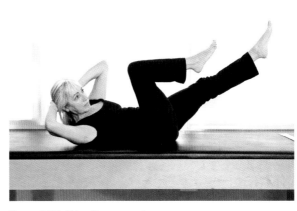

Figure 2.25: Criss-Cross exercise.

Role of the Myofascial System in the Control of Compression

It is important to note that while the deep myofascial system has the ability to create specific joint stability, it cannot perform higher-level activities without the assistance of the superficial system. Use of the superficial myofascial system, balanced by the deep myofascial system, provides the stability needed to perform higher-level tasks such as walking, lifting, and exercising. The superficial myofascial system contributes to these activities by creating stability that is developed via compression.

While the term *compression* might send shivers down your spine as a Pilates teacher or practitioner (since we rarely strive for "compression" during our exercises), it is a balanced or, as Levin and Martin refer to it, a "floating" compression (Schleip 2012) and not a hard-core compressive strategy that we are aiming for. We can maintain this floating compression because the many fascial lines balance each other out, thereby dissipating forces through the system rather than concentrating this force all in one area. Thus the body does not simply function like a stack of blocks that are compressed by gravity: it operates more like a suspension bridge by distributing these forces to create this sense of suspension or floating compression. Compression via activation of the superficial myofascial chains, combined with the decompressive stability generated by the deep myofascial system, provides us with that higher level of stability required to perform tasks such as lifting our children or a heavy bag of groceries, or more challenging Pilates exercises.

Because the superficial muscles tend to be larger and generate higher levels of force, contraction of the superficial myofascial system increases compression on the joints, while activation of the deep myofascial system gives us joint stability without necessarily imposing increased compression upon the joints. The combined action of these two myofascial systems provides us with the right amount of compression or control required for the task in hand without our joints and soft tissues succumbing to the stresses of compression, rotation, and/or tension.

Let's consider these concepts in various Pilates exercises. During Bilateral Leg Lifts (Lower Lift with knees bent) on the cadillac (Figure 2.26(a)), holding the poles over the head, we activate the TVA and deep myofascial system while maintaining neutral alignment of the TPC, and thereby stabilize without over-compression of the spine. More superficially, the obliques and rectus abdominis provide a higher level of activation and compress the internal contents to provide stability of the TPC throughout the movement. In Kneeling Side Kicks (Figure 2.26(b)), we are in a different plane of gravity, but the same mechanism applies. The deep myofascial system of the core maintains stabilization and elongation, while the superficial core (obliques, rectus abdominis, erector spinae, and quadratus lumborum) provide the appropriate amounts of additional support around the TPC.

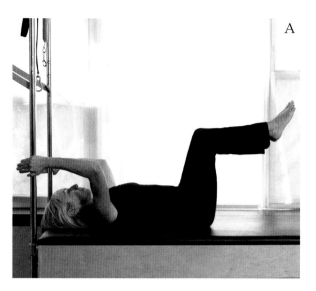

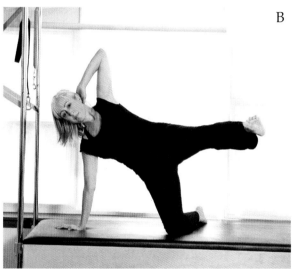

Figure 2.26: (a) Bilateral Leg Lift on the cadillac. (b) Kneeling Side Kicks.

Restore Balance

Developing balance between the deep and superficial myofascial systems is part of an integrative approach to achieving core stability. Non-optimal levels of compression (i.e., too much compression for the task in hand and/or too much compression for too long a period of time) result from the lack of balance between the systems. Incorporating the Pilates principles to restore balance and using the appropriate exercise progressions will help you develop a core-efficient strategy that supports your health and fitness goals.

What is the right amount of compression?

There are three things we are striving for when we talk about compression as part of an optimal strategy of core stabilization:

1. **Feed-forward activation of the deep myofascial system.** Recall that one of the main differentiators between the deep and superficial myofascial systems is that the deep myofascial system is a feed-forward system, meaning these muscles contract prior to the superficial muscles. We want the superficial myofascial system to contract after the deep myofascial system. This is why it is imperative to ensure proper activation of the deep myofascial system during exercise: it stabilizes, decompresses, and keeps the joints from being over-compressed by contraction of the superficial myofascial system during loading.

2. **Focus on precision.** Again, we aim to use the right amount of muscle contraction for the task in hand, and so we need to be specific about how we are performing or teaching exercise. For example, during Leg Circles we want the deep hip muscles (primarily the psoas and deep hip rotators) preferentially activating in order to control and center the femoral head in the acetabulum as the rest of the hip muscles perform the actual movement of the leg (Figure 2.27(a)). If we are not specific with this exercise, the superficial muscles (rectus femoris and TFL) can easily take over (you know that "hip flexor gripping" feeling) and disrupt the optimal axis of rotation, causing hip tightness, grinding, and/or excessive joint compression (Figure 2.27(b)). Over time, this non-optimal strategy can lead to hip impingements, labral tears, and eventually degenerative joint disease.

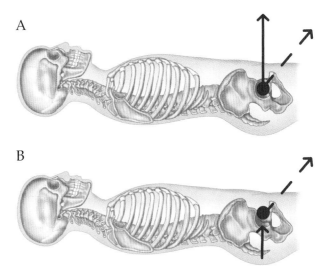

Figure 2.27: (a) With optimal balance between the deep and superficial muscles, the femoral head is controlled within the acetabulum as the leg is lowered during hip flexion. (b) When there is loss of balance between the deep and superficial muscles, the hip joint is not controlled, resulting in an anterior positioning of the femoral head within the acetabulum as the leg is lowered.

3. **Following contraction with relaxation.** A big component of developing an efficient core stabilization strategy is having the ability to turn muscles off or relax them when they are not needed. One of the major problems with muscle inhibition (loss of optimal activation and coordination of the muscle) of the deeper muscles is the subsequent compensation by, and overuse of, the superficial myofascial system as a primary means of stabilization. It is these muscles that tend to become chronically overactive and hypertonic. If the function of the deep myofascial system is not restored, the superficial muscles remain very active and become increasingly resistant to letting go or turning off. Studies have demonstrated that individuals with chronic low back pain, for example, activate their superficial muscles before their deep muscles and do not relax them as easily as they turned them on (Jacobs et al. 2011 and Radebold

et al. 2001). This becomes a significant and common problem because of the long-term compressive forces being placed on the joints. It is important to remember in your training, rehabilitation, and performance that the concept of relaxing your muscles—in other words, getting your nervous system to turn the muscles off when you do not need them—is just as important as your ability to contract them.

Learn to Relax

For many of us, especially those with chronic myofascial tension or hypertonicity, learning to relax our muscles is just as important for the development of an efficient core stabilization strategy as learning when to contract them. In retraining the core, teach your nervous system how to activate the deep myofascial system and coordinate this with breathing prior to activating the superficial myofascial system. The Pilates principles of Concentration (Awareness), Precision, and Breath are especially useful in releasing hypertonic areas and promoting overall relaxation between exercises as well as after the session.

Myofascial Response in Dysfunction

Another differentiating factor of the deep and superficial myofascial systems is their response to trauma and/or injury (Table 1). While there can be variations in response, when there is injury, trauma, and/or inflammation there is often inhibition and atrophy of the deep myofascial system. In response to this, the superficial myofascial system becomes overactive and often hypertonic; this is a central nervous system-mediated reaction to compensate for the loss of joint stability and/or reduce further injury to the joint or soft tissue structures. Although it is a desirable response in the acute phases of an injury, it becomes a problem when there is long-term perpetuation of this muscle imbalance and the muscles contract too much, contract too soon, and/or do not fully disengage (relax) when they are not needed. This is a common reason we experience areas of chronic tightness in our muscles and subsequent over-compression and/or non-optimal positioning of our joints.

The chronic myofascial tightness and joint stiffness we are experiencing is over-activity of the superficial myofascial system and often over-compression, since the myofascial systems are not balanced in their activity. Over time, this compensatory strategy will lead to many of our chronic myofascial tightness and muscle imbalances, which in turn often lead directly to dysfunctional postural and movement patterns, and eventually pain and degenerative soft tissue and/or joint disease. We will delve further into these altered stabilization strategies and compensatory patterns in a later chapter on core dysfunction.

Conclusion

Whether we are exercising, working, or performing activities of daily life, optimal function is predicated on the development of TPC (core) control within our body. Functional control of the TPC is developed by collaboration between the nervous, osseoligamentous, and myofascial systems. We increase our ability to maintain the efficient posture and movement required for life when these systems are functioning optimally— that is, the nervous system receives accurate information and thus provides the right command, the ligamentous system provides proper joint support, the deep myosfascial system pre-activates to stabilize and control the joints, and the superficial myofascial system adds higher levels of control and movement.

We described how efficient posture and movement can only be achieved when there is balance between the two myofascial systems. We should be able to preferentially activate the deep myofascial system to provide joint stability and then recruit the superficial system to create additional stability as required and develop optimal movement patterns. During our Pilates training, we should always strive for balance within our myofascial systems. Balance creates the proper amounts of stabilizing joint compression and decompression required for performing lower-level activities (such as maintaining good posture, walking, and bending) as well as controlling higher-level activities (such as lifting and sports). When we achieve balance between the two systems, we create smooth, integrated, and coordinated posture and movement—that is, we are developing a strategy for health and vitality.

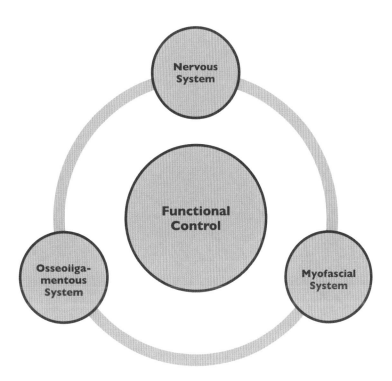

Figure 2.28: Functional control of the TPC is developed by collaboration between the nervous, osseoligamentous, and myofascial systems.

Developing Core Stability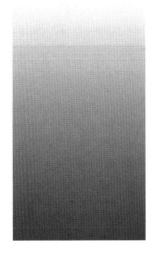

In the last chapter we discussed the deep and superficial muscles of the core and outlined how tensegrity modulates both decompressive and compressive forces in the myofascial system, collectively creating stability of the TPC. In this chapter we will expand upon how the nervous system develops optimal TPC (core) stabilization.

At the most fundamental level, the primary function of the core muscles is stabilization of the trunk, spine, and pelvis. Stabilization allows us to maintain both optimal alignment of our joints and an optimal axis of rotation throughout motion. Whether we are holding a static position such as the Plank or moving through more dynamic exercises like the rolling or twisting patterns, core stability is what allows us to maintain optimal joint alignment while being able to safely express our range of motion (Figure 3.1).

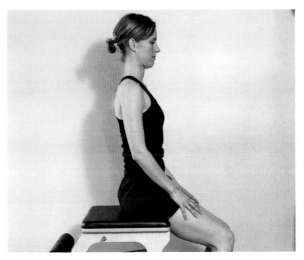 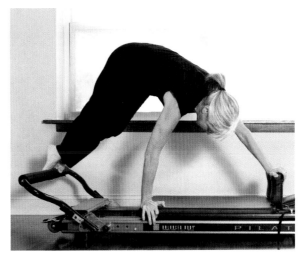

Figure 3.1: Core stabilization is required whether holding a static position, such as sitting, or performing a dynamic exercise on the reformer.

In this chapter we explore:

• The definition of core stability
• How we develop an optimal core stabilization strategy
• The difference between using a low-level versus a high-level stabilization strategy
• The role of control in the development of core stability

We will also discuss the role that abdominal hollowing and bracing play in recruiting the core muscles and demonstrate effective methods for improving core activation during Pilates sessions. In the exercise section we expand on these concepts and demonstrate how to develop and progress an optimal stabilization strategy so that your core functions at a high level whether you are exercising or performing daily life activities.

Defining Stability

The complex and myriad nature of life's tasks requires a core stabilization strategy that is efficient and adaptable. We define *core stability* as "the right amount of control at the right time for the task in hand" (Osar 2013). Another way of saying this is that the individual possesses efficient control of their posture and movement as they perform their functional tasks. The point is not whether a person can stabilize their core, but whether they are using the best strategy for the task they are performing (Figure 3.2).

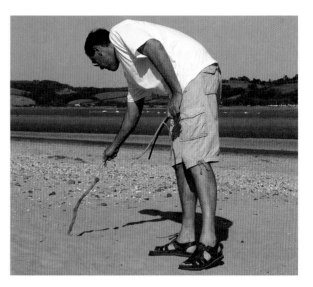

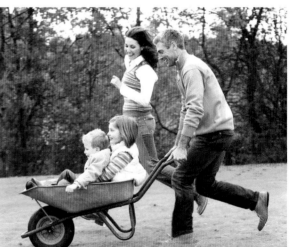

Figure 3.2: Whether bending forward to dig in the sand or lifting a loaded wheelbarrow full of kids, we require core stability for the activity to be smooth, coordinated, and controlled. However, a different level of effort or intensity is required to adequately support the trunk, spine, and pelvis in each of these activities. Using the same effort—for example, overly bracing the core—for every activity is one of the hallmarks of an inefficient strategy that leads to the development of faulty posture, movement, and pain syndromes.

Let's look at this concept of core stabilization by comparing the Hamstring Curls on the Long Box (Figure 3.3(a)) with the Long Stretch (Figure 3.3(b)) performed on the reformer; both patterns are excellent for developing optimal core stability. Because the model is supported on the long box and only lifting one leg at a time, the Hamstring Curls requires less overall muscle activation than the Plank pattern. The same strategy will be used for stabilization in each pattern—the deep myofascial system will preferentially activate, and the superficial myofascial system will be recruited as required; however, the intensity will vary based upon the demands of the exercise.

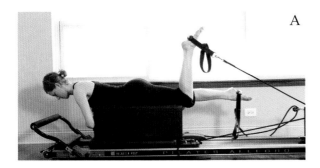

A

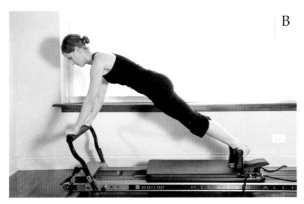

B

Figure 3.3: (a) Hamstring Curls on the Long Box; (b) Plank/Long Stretch on the Reformer.

The important concept here is that we need efficient low-level stabilization (which is required for low-level tasks) as well as high-level stabilization strategies. Low-level tasks—such as quiet standing and sitting, bending, rotating, breathing while at rest, and walking at an even pace—should not require a significant level of muscular effort to stabilize. Tasks that have higher demands, and thus require higher levels of stabilization, include walking at a rapid pace, up an incline, or up stairs; running; breathing heavily while exercising; lifting anything with weight that challenges the individual; and rotating the trunk rapidly to throw a ball or swing a golf club.

This is why it is just as important to teach an individual to control lower-demand exercises, such as the Hamstring Curls (Figure 3.3(a)), as it is to develop control of higher-level patterns, such as the Plank. Many individuals who experience chronic tightness and issues like low back pain with sitting, standing, or bending tend to use a high-level strategy for these low-level tasks. In other words, they over-recruit their superficial myofascial system for tasks that should not require a high level of activity.

To understand why this occurs, we must consider our nervous system's response to stress. When there is an injury, trauma, and/or joint inflammation, the deep myofascial system tends to become preferentially inhibited. Once inhibited, this system is unable to provide the optimal proprioceptive feedback to the CNS required for activating and coordinating the myofascial systems to control the joints during posture and movement. Not wanting to incur additional joint or soft tissue stress, the nervous system compensates by increasing activation of the superficial myofascial system. In the short term, this strategy does indeed provide a level of control and protection of the joints and soft tissues.

The problem arises when this becomes the default strategy for stabilization, meaning we use it all the time, even for relative low-level tasks. This can be equated to the volume button being broken on your radio and stuck on the loudest volume, with no way to adjust the level; it is just always on high.

A significant problem occurs when a client is advanced too quickly through the Pilates repertoire, before they have learned how to optimally pre-activate their deep myofascial system and develop sufficient strength and endurance to stabilize it under increasing loads: the client will inevitably succumb to a higher-level bracing strategy and tend to overuse the superficial myofascial system.

Let's return to our example of the Plank position on the reformer in the Long Stretch (Figure 3.4). As mentioned earlier, each exercise pattern requires a level of stabilization effort that is appropriately matched to its intensity. It is common for a new Pilates student, or one who has been experiencing chronic tightness or pain in their core muscles, to struggle to stabilize their core without the appropriate level of muscle activation or without losing control of their neutral spine alignment. You may note that they shift their pelvis, flatten their back, and/or over-contract and grip their superficial hip flexors as they initiate hip flexion.

Fortunately, the Pilates repertoire offers many opportunities to expose these non-optimal strategies for stabilization. Consider Leg Springs on the reformer. New students are surprised at how challenging it is to manage a relatively low load without compensation. "This is harder than it looks," they will say as they struggle to locate the deeper control required for smooth execution of Leg Circles and Frogs. But only by performing such seemingly "easy" exercises do beginning students learn to "turn down the volume" (be that in their mind and/or in the superficial muscles) enough to access the muscles of the deep core. Were these same students to attempt an exercise such as the Double-Leg Circles on the mat, without first developing the deep core stability they would likely over-arch and possibly strain the low back, flare the ribs, clench the glutes, and brace and/or "pooch" the abdominals as the hip flexors and low back attempt to hold things together. The way we move in Pilates reveals the strategies we use to stabilize the core during daily activities. The beauty of the Pilates repertoire is that we

can help people identify and develop a more optimal strategy.

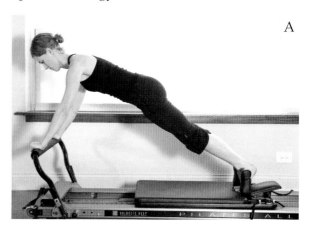

A

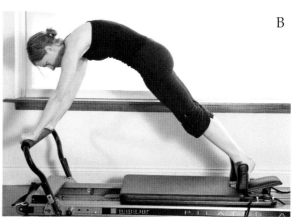

B

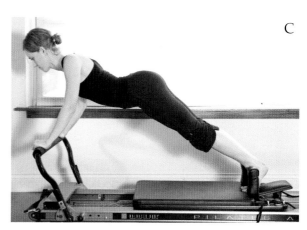

C

Figure 3.4: (a) Neutral alignment and control in the Plank position. (b) Over-recruitment of the superficial abdominal muscles to stabilize the position. (c) Over-recruitment of the hip flexors and erector spinae muscles. The last two are examples of non-optimal recruitment strategies that will lead to and/or perpetuate low back, pelvis and hip dysfunction.

Case Study

Figure 3.5 shows a client who presented with low back pain whenever he stood or walked for any period of time. He had no pain while sitting at his desk working. His physical activity included playing soccer once a week. Notice the significant hypertonicity in his erector spinae muscles around his thoracolumbar region. Why does an individual who sits at a desk all day and only exercises sporadically exhibit such significant tone in these muscles? Observe this individual's sitting posture. Notice how he is sitting in a posterior pelvic tilt, with excessive flexion in both the lumbar and thoracic regions of the spine. This is a non-optimal strategy for sitting that will create increased stress upon the discs and soft tissues of the spine.

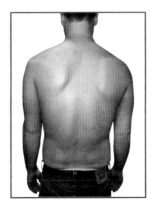

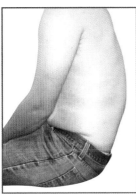

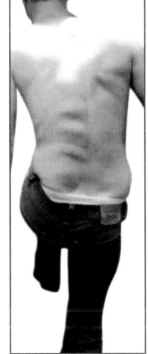

Figure 3.5: Low back pain: the result of non-optimal stabilization strategies.

Next, note what happens when this individual stands on one leg. Notice the increased activity in his erector spinae muscles as he attempts to balance or stabilize himself. This is a classic example of using a high-level strategy for a relatively low-level task. This also explains why he experiences increased discomfort when he stands or walks: he has to excessively use his superficial myofascial system to create a level of optimal stability to perform the required task. The goal with this individual is to teach him an improved stabilization strategy that helps him better align and center his trunk as well as his lower extremities. Additionally, he must be able to support himself in a proper posture, without excessively gripping or over-contracting his superficial myofascial system.

Pilates is about creating options for the body. It is important to have a variety of stabilizing strategies available to us and to be able to spontaneously employ the most functional strategy for the task in hand. The right strategy comes from having the deep and superficial myofascial systems working synergistically, where the deep system controls segmental motion and the superficial system adds a higher level of control as required. Developing the balance between these two is what functional core stability is all about.

Develop an Optimal Core Strategy
Efficient posture and movement come from having an optimal core stabilization strategy for the task in hand. This strategy should be adaptable in order to meet the demands of the task without overloading any one region of the body, which often occurs with non-optimal strategies. Being disciplined in applying the Pilates principles helps develop a core stabilization strategy that promotes control and adaptability to meet the demands of sport, occupations, and life.

Developing an Efficient Core Stabilization Strategy

In the previous section we defined stability and noted that to have optimal stabilization, we must be able to vary our strategy based on the demands of the task. In this section we will now look at the methods that enable us to produce an adaptable and efficient core stabilization strategy.

Optimal core stability is developed through a combination of pressure and tension. When we have an integrated and balanced system, we can control and/or resist excessive shear, tensile, rotary, and compressive forces through pressure and tension. Without this control, our movement could be creating repetitive traumas and over-compression of our joints every time we change positions, lift something, or accelerate/decelerate our body.

In this section we discuss the following:

- The forces that the core has to stabilize against during exercise and life
- The role of intra-abdominal pressure in the development of core stability
- How breathing and muscle activation develops pressure and tension to provide efficient core control

Stabilization Against Forces on the Body

Each day, and with virtually every single movement in life, our body is subject to forces that if left unchecked, would create damaging stresses upon our soft tissue and joints (Figure 3.6). An efficient core stabilization strategy protects our joints from excessive tensile, compressive, rotary, and shear forces while helping us maintain optimal posture and movement patterns (Figure 3.7). Developing an efficient stabilization strategy allows flexibility of the thorax, spine, and pelvis, and provides the support required to effortlessly perform the relatively simple tasks of breathing and walking, or the incredibly coordinated tasks of dancing or playing sports.

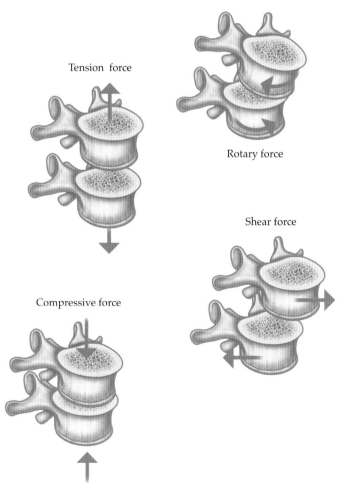

Tension force

Rotary force

Shear force

Compressive force

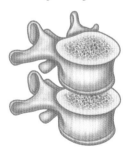

Original alignment

Figure 3.6: Examples of the forces that our joints are subjected to during posture and movement. An optimal core stabilization strategy provides us with control against these forces.

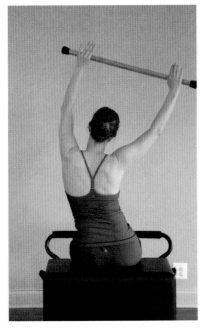
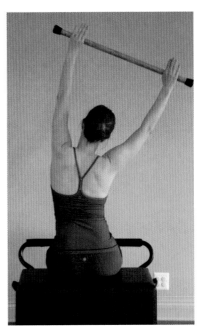
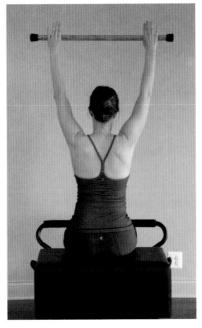
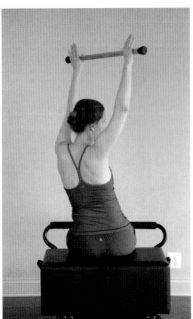
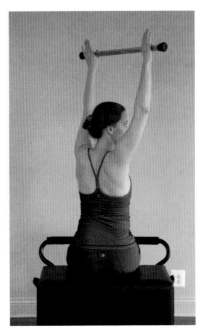

Figure 3.7: Note the compressive shear forces on the spine in the images to the left, compared with the decompressive stability seen in the same motions to the right.

Intra-abdominal Pressure

Even in grade school biology classes, we learned the importance of breathing for our overall health. Respiration is the method by which our pulmonary and cardiovascular systems take in oxygen and distribute it throughout the body; as we breathe out, the same systems help remove waste products.

However, in the light of recent research, we can now say with confidence that optimal breathing has another significant role in our body—stabilization. Research has demonstrated that the diaphragm has the dual role of supporting both respiration and posture (Hodges and Gandevia 2000). While the actions of the TVA and diaphragm oppose each other (contraction of the diaphragm increases the volume of the thoracic cavity, whereas contraction of the TVA decreases the volume), both muscles are constantly contributing to respiration and postural control and the development of intra-abdominal pressure (IAP).

Developing IAP is one of the most important strategies for resisting forces, particularly compressive forces, that are placed on the spine, thorax, and pelvis. These compressive forces (Figure 3.8) include:

• The downward-directed forces of gravity
• Our own body weight
• The passive myofascial tension while at rest, and the active tension with active contraction
• Any external load we place on our body when lifting
• Forces that are transmitted to the body when our foot hits the ground (the force of the foot hitting the ground creates an equal and opposite force that travels back up the body and into our core)

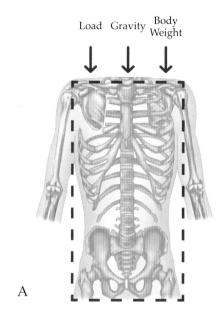

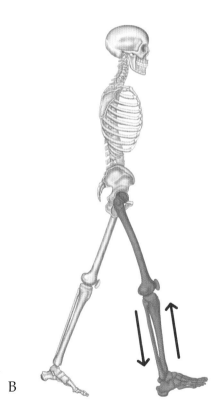

Figure 3.8: (a) Forces—including gravity, external loads, and our body weight—work to compress our spine. (b) Ground reaction forces—forces that are generated from the impact of our foot hitting the ground—are controlled by a well-functioning core.

Our body is regularly subjected to compressive forces that we are fully capable of resisting when we have an efficient stabilization strategy. Intra-abdominal pressure is the best strategy for negotiating these compressive forces; additionally, it enables us to stabilize our core while simultaneously decompressing our joints. This allows us to develop posture and movement that is smooth, coordinated, and well controlled.

Create Core Stability

Intra-abdominal pressure is the part of our core stabilization strategy that enables us to simultaneously stabilize *and* decompress the TPC. This gives us the ability to create core stability while diminishing the stresses of being over-compressed. Improving our awareness in how we breathe, along with ensuring optimal use of three-dimensional breathing, is one of the most effective strategies we have found for improving posture and movement while releasing chronic myofascial tension.

You can visualize IAP in the following way. Imagine blowing up a sturdy stability ball inside a cardboard box. Imagine that this box is also filled with stacked eggs. When the ball is blown up and firm, it dramatically increases the stability of the box (i.e., it improves its resistance to being crushed). You could essentially sit on the box without crushing it or the eggs. This occurs because of the internal pressure and outward stability generated by the ball.

Now imagine that the thoracic and pelvic cavities are the box surrounding the eggs and that the pressure built up inside these cavities (intra-abdominal pressure) is the stability ball. In this model, the pressure generated inside the cavities stabilizes the spine and prevents the viscera (the eggs) from being overly compressed by a combination of the forces we discussed earlier (Figure 3.9).

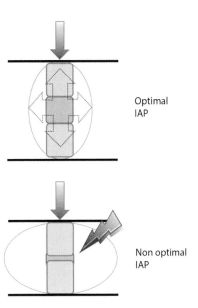

Figure 3.9: When a state of optimal intra-abdominal pressure (IAP) exists, the body is able to resist compressive forces, and our joints are well protected (top image). However, when we lose the ability to generate intra-abdominal pressure, or the compressive load is greater than we are able to handle, our joints become over-compressed (bottom image). This is why it becomes imperative to improve breathing and achieve a balance between the deep and superficial muscle systems; this helps the individual develop the proper intra-abdominal pressure to sustain optimal alignment and control throughout exercise and life activities.

IAP provides stability and resistance to both external forces (gravity, bodyweight, and ground reaction forces) and internal myofascial tension (force created by the passive and active tension in the muscles). How does the body generate the optimum levels of pressure inside the thoracic and abdominal cavities? It is developed through optimal respiration in much the same way a hydraulic press operates. The mouth and throat—or more specifically, the vocal folds—can be equated to the intake area of a hydraulic press, and the thoracic and abdominal regions can be equated to the output area. The diaphragm and intercostal muscles contract to move moistened air (the compressed liquid in our body) into the trachea through the vocal folds, where it causes an increase in the pressure within the thoracic and abdominal areas, creating a pressurized and stable trunk, spine, and pelvis (Figure 3.10).

How do we manage to maintain intra-abdominal pressure during expiration? The activity of the abdominal muscles (contraction of the TVA) and passive shortening of the myofascial structures around the thorax, as well as the decreasing diameter of the thoracic and abdominal cavities during exhalation, maintain a relatively constant stabilizing pressure as the diaphragm ascends. In this manner, we can maintain IAP throughout the entire respiratory cycle.

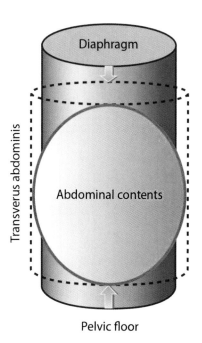

Figure 3.10: Generation of the optimum levels of pressure inside the thoracic and abdominal cavities.

As discussed, IAP functions to resist the downward-directed forces of gravity, the bodyweight and myofascial pull, and any external loads, as well as the upward-directed ground reaction forces that are generated as the foot hits the ground and the ground pushes back, sending force back up through the spine (Figure 3.9, see page 57). This has an effect of simultaneously stabilizing the trunk, spine, and pelvis and decompressing these areas. When we have a non-optimal strategy, these forces place a compressive load on the spine and lead to many of the common spinal-related issues we experience, such as disc bulges/herniations and degenerative osteoarthritic changes of the trunk, spine, pelvis, and hips.

Without IAP to decrease the downward pressure generated within the thoracic and abdominal cavities, increased pressure is directed into the pelvic cavity. This places increased stress on the pelvic floor and, over time, potentially increases the risk and/or perpetuation of urinary incontinence. Subsequently, many individuals will over-contract their hip muscles to help support the pelvic floor, thereby creating tightness in the hips and developing non-optimal posture and movement habits.

Certain Pilates exercises—like Teaser, Roll-Up, and Double-Leg Lift (Figure 3.11)—that encourage flexion or "imprinting" of the spine particularly require the use of IAP for stabilization, as there is the potential for these patterns to increase the compressive forces on the spine and into the pelvic region. If performed without an effective stabilization strategy, these exercises push the abdominal contents inferiorly, increasing intra-pelvic pressure and placing increased pressure on the spine, lower abdominal wall, and pelvic floor. This is a common contributing cause of urinary continence, since the pelvic floor is not designed to resist all that downward pressure on its own. When the pressures are managed through the synergistic effects of the diaphragms (respiratory and urogenital) and the abdominal muscles, there is less pressure placed upon the pelvic floor and it can optimally control bowel and bladder function.

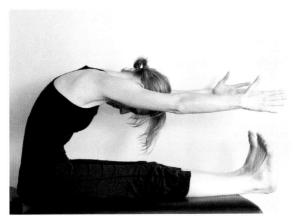
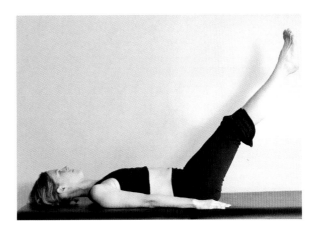

Figure 3.11: (a) Roll-Up. (b) Double-Leg Lift.

To avoid the potentially damaging effects of this downward IAP on the pelvic floor, keep an eye out for "bulging" abdominals during these patterns. You can always use bands and springs for support and to help lighten the load. Keeping the front ribcage open on exercises such as the Roll-Up is another way to prevent downward pressure on the pelvic floor (Calais-Garmain and Raison 2010). This action gently lifts the viscera up (as opposed to pushing them down towards the perineum, which is common during abdominal bracing). You might also imagine a net or harness gently lifting the intestines and other organs up towards your ribcage (not forcefully; imagine the lift is less than an inch) during these patterns; this will activate the deep abdominal wall and pelvic floor first and ensure the proper support.

Breath is also key. Monitoring yourself for a fluid breath and an open throat throughout the exercise is essential to avoid harmful patterns. Pay special attention during exercises like the Hundred! Forceful exhalation *can* damage the perineum as a result of the downward movement of the abdominal contents (Calais-Garmain and Raison 2010). Stay safe by lowering the load (feet down or in table top position), and heeding the kinesthetic milestones (such as maintaining your deep core connection) that are discussed in the last chapter of this book.

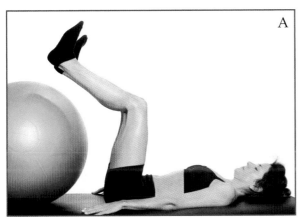
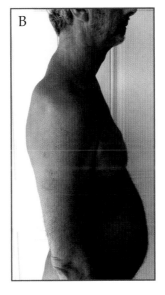

Figure 3.12: (a) Be sure to activate the deep abdominal wall and pelvic floor and coordinate this with controlled breathing for optimal spinal and pelvic support. (b) Note the abdominal bulging or distension in this individual with a non-optimal core stabilization strategy.

In figure 3.12(b) (page 59) note the abdominal bulging or distension which occurs when there is excessive downward pressure that is not controlled by a proper intra-abdominal pressure strategy. Be sure to activate the deep abdominal wall and pelvic floor and coordinate this with controlled breathing for optimal spinal and pelvic support.

To efficiently move our body and to live life without resorting to compressive types of strategy, it is essential that we breathe correctly to activate the deep myofascial system and develop the IAP required for posture and movement. Next we will look at a method for developing three-dimensional breathing and creating intra-abdominal pressure, which is required to stabilize our trunk, spine, and pelvis. We will demonstrate how to coordinate respiration with activation of the deep myofascial system in developing a more efficient core stabilization strategy. This strategy includes and promotes alignment and Centering, Concentration, Breath, Control, Precision, and eventually Flow. In essence, this strategy incorporates all the Pilates principles into one simple exercise progression.

Developing Three-Dimensional Breathing and Activating the Deep Myofascial System

Developing awareness and control of neutral alignment is an extremely important component of developing a more efficient core stabilization strategy. *Neutral posture* is where the joints are in a relatively low-load position, which can also be considered a physiologically efficient position because it requires the least amount of effort to maintain. One of the things we will look at later is how increased myofascial activity is required for holding non-optimal posture and for the resultant movement patterns. Neutral posture has also been shown to be one of the best positions for

activating the muscles of the deep myofascial system, such as the transversus abdominis and pelvic floor (Richardson et al. 2004).

We have also found that because so many individuals have developed non-optimal or compensated postural strategies, neutral posture is the most challenging position to find and control for most people. Therefore our goal is to align the body in a way that helps the individual achieve their most neutral posture. In the case of those who have had chronic postural compensations and for whom it is challenging to achieve neutral alignment, we will position such individuals in a way that best helps them approximate a neutral spine while relaxing their superficial myofascial system.

Although various positions can be used, we will begin in a supine position. The goal is to arrange the body in a way that supports neutral alignment of the head, trunk, spine, and pelvis. The supine position is also one of the earliest positions in which we first establish joint alignment, breathing, and core control. Thus it can be very beneficial to return to the "Happy Baby" pose to re-establish and promote optimal core function (Figure 3.13).

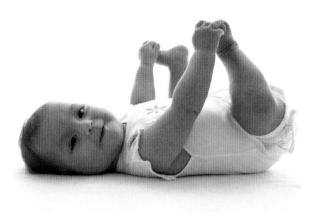

Figure 3.13: Happy Baby pose.

Alignment for Optimal Breathing

To achieve optimal respiration as well as core activation, the joints of the head, neck, and TPC should be neutrally aligned and centered over the top of each other. This position will facilitate joint alignment and the muscle activation patterns required for ideal respiration and stabilization.

The objective is to align the TPC in such a way that the head is neutrally positioned in line with the trunk. In standing, when viewed from the side, ideally a plumb line should drop through the middle of the ear, the bodies of the lower cervical vertebrae, and then just anterior to the mid-thoracic spine. The goal is to align yourself or your clients in a similar position, ensuring that the head is level when viewed from the side. This position is vital, since you want the head and neck positioned so that the activity of the deep neck flexors is optimized and they can properly assist with neck stability while minimizing the use of the scalenes and sternocleidomastoid muscles, two muscles that are most responsible for forward-head and forward-neck postures.

The thorax should be positioned so that the inferior thoracic opening (bottom of the ribcage) opens up towards the pelvis. The spine should be straight when viewed from the front and back, and retain its natural curves when viewed from the side. The pelvis should in neutral alignment under the thorax and positioned symmetrically over the femoral heads.

It is unlikely that individuals with significant forward-head posture will be able to achieve the proper position when supine, shown in Figure 3.14, however. In this case, supports can be used under the head, neck, and/or shoulders to help place the individual in a way that allows them to be as neutral as possible,

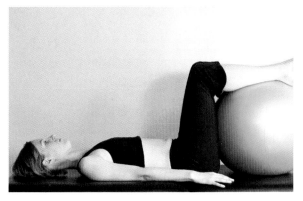

Figure 3.14: (a) Proper alignment of the head and TPC in standing. (b) Proper alignment in the supine position. Note the similarity to the Happy Baby position discussed earlier, which supports proper respiration and muscle activation.

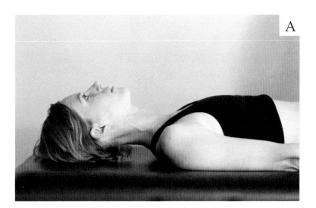

A

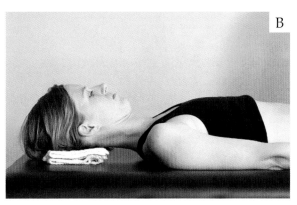

B

Figure 3.15: Towel support or bolster support can be used to align the head in individuals with suboccipital extension and/or increased thoracic kyphosis: (a) non-optimal; (b) optimal.

with the least amount of stress placed on their joints (Figure 3.15). The legs will be elevated so that the hips and knees are flexed and the pelvis remains neutral.

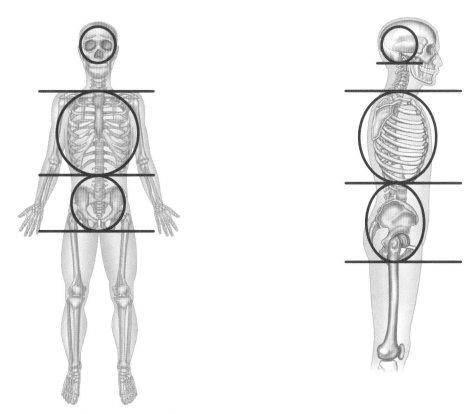

Figure 3.16: The transverse fascia covering the thoracic inlet, the respiratory diaphragm, and the urogenital diaphragm (pelvic floor). With optimal alignment of the head, neck and TPC, these three diaphragms function as both pressure regulators and suspensory support systems.

In addition to aligning the bones of the core, trunk, spine, and pelvis, the neutral position allows us to align the three diaphragms of the TPC: the thoracic inlet (transverse fascial layer covering the top of both lungs), the respiratory diaphragm, and the urogenital diaphragm (pelvic floor). Alignment of these diaphragms helps modulate pressures within the different cavities of the body and supports the surrounding organs. Additionally, better alignment of the TPC, and hence the diaphragms, will increase the ability to relax excessive compensatory myofascial tension around the trunk, spine, and pelvis (Figure 3.16).

Loss of optimal TPC alignment can be created by excessive extension at the thoracolumbar junction (TLJ)—the region where the lower ribcage and thoracic spine join the lumbar spine (Figure 3.17). In this position, the diaphragms are not aligned to support proper breathing or pressure regulation. This posture also makes it impossible to achieve optimal transversus abdominis activation and places increased pressure upon the pelvic floor.

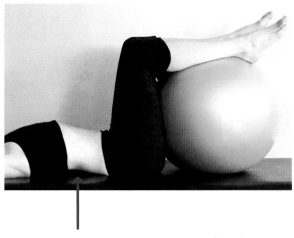

Figure 3.17: Loss of optimal TPC alignment where the inferior ribcage is flared and not aligned with the pelvis.

Motion of the Thorax and Diaphragm During Respiration

Whether you are a Pilates enthusiast or instructor, understanding and recognizing what constitutes ideal respiratory mechanics is important, because this lays the foundation for developing efficient core stabilization. We will discuss these ideal mechanics as well as some of the methods we have found to be successful in developing or restoring optimal respiration in our clients and patients. Our most important goal is to improve the mechanics of respiration and coordinate this with activation of the deep myofascial system. We are not striving for perfection, but attempting to move towards establishing a more efficient strategy for the individual. We have repeatedly seen dramatic improvements in posture, reduction of chronic muscle tension, and increases in strength when individuals discover how to breathe and coordinate activation of their deep myofascial system.

One important note regarding breathing: improving three-dimensional breathing can create a profound effect in individuals who have not been breathing efficiently. For these individuals, it is important to start slowly rather than attempting to improve their mechanics too quickly; do not force breathing. Bring their awareness to an area where they may not be breathing well, encourage three-dimensional breathing with light palpation, and start with fewer breaths (one to three at a time). Then let them return to their normal strategy of breathing between cycles. Light-headedness or dizziness can occur as a client begins developing a more efficient breathing strategy; if this occurs, have the client stop immediately and return to their normal rate and depth of breathing until they feel back to normal.

- **Inhalation**: As we inhale, contraction of the diaphragm and intercostals causes the ribs to open, in a way similar to the opening of an accordion. The diaphragm moves inferiorly, relative to its resting position in the mid-thorax, pushing the abdominal contents down towards the pelvis: the abdomen expands therefore during inhalation. Contraction of the sternocleidomastoid, scalenes, and pectoralis minor help elevate the sternum and upper ribs, contributing to an anteroposterior (front-to-back) expansion of the thorax. The intercostals and levator costarum contribute to increasing the intercostal space (i.e., space between the ribs), aiding in the expansion of the thorax (Figures 3.18–20). At the posterior aspect of the ribcage, the serratus posterior superior elevates the upper ribs, and the serratus posterior inferior and quadratus lumborum lower the lower ribs, expanding the superior-to-inferior dimensions of the thorax.

While at rest and performing quiet breathing, the abdominal muscles should be relatively relaxed to allow for ease of motion within the thorax. During exercise or labored breathing, the abdominal muscles resist the action of the transversus abdominis and intercostals; this action functions to improve trunk, spine, and pelvic stability.

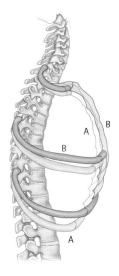

Figure 3.18: Position of the sternum and ribs at the end of exhalation (A); with inhalation both the sternum and ribs elevate to increase the anterior to posterior dimensions of the thorax (B).

• **Exhalation:** During exhalation there is essentially a reversal of the actions that occur during inhalation. The diaphragm eccentrically contracts (elongates) and ascends into the thorax. The intercostal spaces decrease and the ribs approximate as the sternum descends because of the relaxation (actually an eccentric contraction) of the muscles controlling them, which decreases the volume of the thorax.

The thoracic volume also decreases as a result of the relative passive tension created in the myofascial structures surrounding the TPC during inspiration, and because of the change in intra-thoracic pressure (the internal pressure being greater inside the thoracic cavity immediately following the inhalation), which reflexively facilitates expiration.

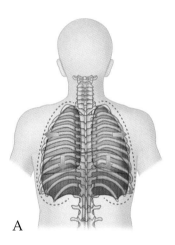
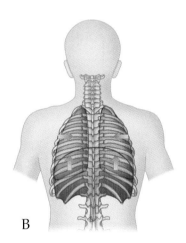

Figure 3.19: Posterior aspect of the TPC during inspiration (a) and expiration (b).

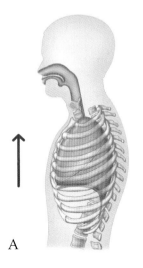
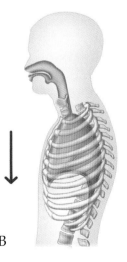

Figure 3.20: (a) As the individual breathes in, the sternum rotates upward, there is an increase in the intercostal spaces, and the diaphragm descends, thereby increasing the dimensions of the thorax. (b) During expiration, the diaphragm elevates, the sternum descends, and the intercostal spaces narrow, which collectively decrease the dimensions of the thorax.

The muscles of respiration have been designated in the literature as having either a primary role (i.e., they are most responsible) or an accessory role, meaning they assist the primary muscles, in breathing. While there are definitely muscles that have a more primary role, most of the muscles listed in Table 3.1 play a significant role in developing an optimal resting or quiet breathing strategy, regardless of their categorization.

Several muscles, including the sternalis and levator costarum, have not been adequately studied, so we do not know their exact functional role in respiratory mechanics or core stabilization. At this time, all we can surmise is that because of their attachments on the thorax, they likely have a role in respiration and therefore in postural control.

Primary Muscles	Accessory Muscles
Diaphragm—respiratory	Sternocleidomastoid
Scalenes—all three divisions	Subclavius
Serratus posterior superior	Pectoralis minor
Serratus posterior inferior	Upper trapezius
Sternalis	Levator scapulae
Transversus thoracis	Serratus anterior
Quadratus lumborum	Erector spinae
Abdominals	
External intercostals	
Internal intercostals	
Levator costarum—brevis and longus	

Table 3.1: The muscles of respiration.

The muscles most active during quiet respiration are generally listed as primary muscles of respiration. When these muscles become inhibited or their function is altered, there is a dramatic effect on posture and stabilization, as the accessory muscles (primarily the sternocleidomastoid, upper trapezius, levator scapulae, and pectoralis) become overactive to aid respiration. Later on we will look more closely at the roles of muscle inhibition, myofascial hypertonicity, and stress in the manifestation of faulty respiratory mechanics and the development of compensatory stabilization and movement patterns.

Retraining an Optimal Breathing Strategy

Beginning in supine with the legs elevated and supported (similar to the Happy Baby position) is the easiest position for retraining respiration in most individuals. This position serves several roles in retraining optimal breathing:

1. It is the best position in which to achieve neutral alignment of the spine, trunk, and pelvis as well as alignment of the three diaphragms.

2. It is the least stressful position for the joints and discs of the spine, making it easier to facilitate the joint motion required to fully expand the thorax during respiration.

3. The effects of gravity on the spine are at a minimum in this position; thus it helps relax excessive muscle tension that may inhibit optimal expansion of the thorax.

4. The pressure of the floor or surface against the individual's back provides kinesthetic feedback to increase awareness and help the individual self-monitor the position of their head, trunk, spine, and pelvis.

5. It is one of the earliest positions in which we developed optimal breathing and stabilization as children, and thus is familiar to our nervous system.

We will retrain breathing in three separate steps, delineated as the functional ABCs of respiration and stabilization: alignment, breathing, and coordination.

Step 1—Alignment

The individual will elevate their legs so that their hips and knees are both at 90-degree angles. People with stiff or limited hip mobility may require a hip angle slightly greater than 90 degrees, with the knees moved slightly further away from the head. The legs would be resting on a coffee table or chair if at home, but a stability ball can be used in a gym setting (Figure 3.21(a)). However, the narrowness and instability of the ball do not allow the hips to rest in their anatomical position or allow the hip muscles to completely relax, which is why a ball is not ideal and another option for elevating them is preferable. If you are working in an area where no support is available, it is all right to work in the hook-lying position, where the knees are bent and the feet are flat on the floor (Figure 3.21(b)).

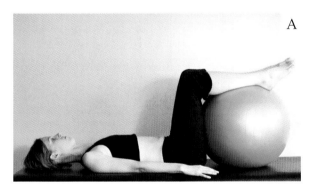

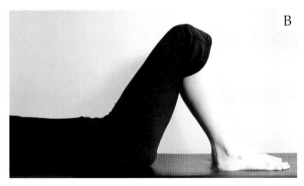

Figure 3.21: (a) Legs supported on a stability ball. (b) Hook lying.

For many individuals, it can be beneficial to release chronic tension around the TPC. Pelvic Tilts and self-myofascial release (SMFR) are two methods for mobilizing the soft tissues around the hips and spine prior to instituting breathing and core activation.

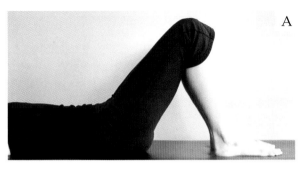

A

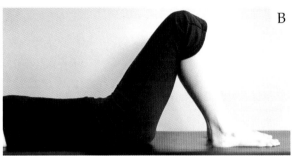

B

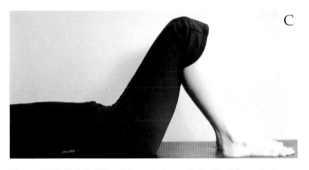

C

Figure 3.22: Pelvic Tilts: (a) posterior pelvic tilt; (b) neutral pelvic alignment; (c) anterior pelvic tilt.

Pelvic Tilts (Figure 3.22) can help reduce myofascial hypertonicity and gripping around the hips and spine, so that the individual is able to achieve more neutral alignment once their legs are in the supported position. The individual is in a relative neutral pelvic position when their anterior superior iliac spines (ASISs) are in the same relative horizontal plane as their pubic symphysis. Pelvic Tilts are a great way to enhance an individual's awareness and to become familiar with the motion of their pelvis. They are also effective in reducing hypertonicity around the hips and spine, while helping to re-establish the pelvis and lumbar spine in a more neutral position.

Soft tissue release with balls and foam rollers (Figure 3.23, see overleaf) can also be extremely beneficial in releasing myofascial restrictions around the thorax, lumbar spine, and/or hips, making it easier to achieve more optimal alignment. SMFR can be especially effective at the thoracolumbar junction (the region between the bottom of the ribcage and beginning of the lumbar spine), where many individuals develop chronic myofascial tension and gripping. This technique can be useful in facilitating more ideal thoracic mobility, which is required to begin breath retraining. Be sure to use caution when performing SMFR over the spine and/or ribs. With individuals who have osteoporosis and/ or have recently had surgery or an acute injury, it is advisable to stay off the bones and remain in the soft tissue structures of the trunk and spine, to avoid creating osseous stress, or even subluxations (malposition of the spine).

Once in the ideal set-up position, with the legs either supported or in hook lying, the individual will perform a series of five to ten alternating anterior and posterior pelvic tilts before coming to rest in the most neutral pelvic position they can find. To monitor this position, have the individual place one hand over their ASIS and, starting from their belly button, slide the other hand down their abdomen until it rests over the pubic symphysis. These two bones should be aligned horizontally with each other.

A

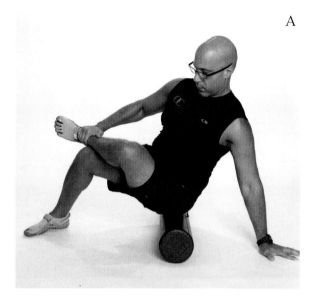

B

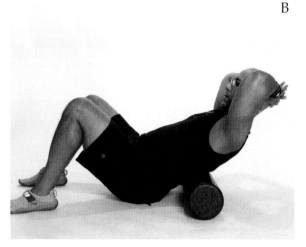

Figure 3.23: Self-myofascial release (SMFR) with a foam roller: (a) hips; (b) thorax.

There are times when simply placing the individual in a position that aligns their joints and soft tissue structures, especially the diaphragms, is enough to decrease overactive components of the myofascial system and naturally facilitate a more ideal breathing pattern. If the individual's system is not too dysfunctional, or the dysfunction has not been there for a long period of time, aligning the joints can improve proprioception and activation of the right muscles, promoting ideal function. Generally, most individuals will require specific retraining and will have to

be guided through exactly how and where to breathe, in order to enhance optimal function.

Step 2—Breathing

Once the individual is optimally aligned, we can begin retraining their breathing. Recall that aligning the bones and soft tissue structures in Step 1 allows the greatest likelihood of developing the proper breathing and muscle activation that is required for the ideal core stabilization. The eventual goal of developing an optimal breathing strategy is to have each region of the TPC contribute to overall respiratory mechanics. *Three-dimensional respiration* refers to the process whereby the entire thorax is involved in the breathing action: in other words, there is superior–inferior (top-to-bottom), lateral (side-to-side), and anteroposterior (front-to-back) expansion of the ribcage during inhalation (Figure 3.24).

A   B   C

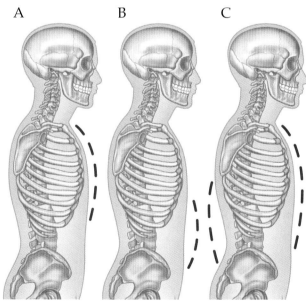

Figure 3.24: Note the non-optimal breathing strategies: (a) predominately apical, or chest; (b) predominately abdominal, or belly. The optimal three-dimensional respiration in image (c) increases the entire thoracic and abdominal cavities, even expanding into the back.

It is often easier to segment out the individual regions (abdominal, costal, and posterolateral) of the thorax during initial breath retraining; generally, the progression moves from easiest (abdominal) to most challenging (posterolateral). An important component of breath retraining is to increase the individual's awareness of the area where they may not have ideal mechanics, so that they can repeat the process on their own. Bringing awareness to our current habits is the most important step in facilitating change, because we are unable to change patterns that we are not aware of.

The best way to begin creating awareness is by becoming familiar with your current breathing strategy. Are you taking a full breath or shallow breaths? Is the breath primarily going into your neck, chest, abdomen, ribcage, or back?

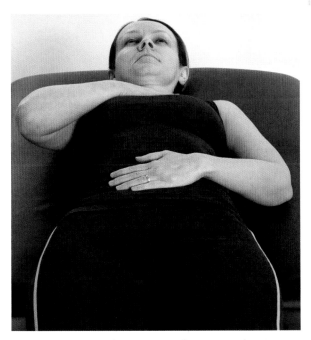

Figure 3.25: Place one hand on your chest and one hand on your abdomen. Which do you feel move more? When breathing optimally, you should feel the hand on your abdomen move first and move more than the hand on the chest.

Next place your hands flat along either side of your lower ribs, just below your chest. Can you feel your ribs open and close, symmetrically, which signifies optimal rib motion during breathing? Now check out your back. Can you feel yourself breathing into the surface you are lying on, indicating that you are achieving optimal movement of the posterior aspect of the diaphragm and expanding the back side of the ribcage?

Focus on a Region
When retraining an optimal breathing strategy, it is often necessary to focus individually on each region (abdominal, costal, posterolateral) to ensure that we are using the proper mechanics and accessing all three regions. This regional focus also helps bring awareness, attention, and purposefulness to the task, which improves performance.

Abdominal Breathing
The first, and generally easiest, place to observe and start retraining is abdominal breathing. To clarify, there is technically no such thing as "abdominal breathing." When the diaphragm contracts, it pushes down on the abdominal contents, and as the abdominal contents are pushed down in the abdominal cavity, we feel expansion of the abdominal region. This is what we are referring to when we say *abdominal breathing*.

To facilitate abdominal breathing and determine whether you are getting optimal diaphragmatic contraction, place your fingers inside both ASISs (Figure 3.26). Now take a breath in and see if you can feel your lower abdominal wall push out into your fingers. An optimal abdominal breath, facilitated by a strong contraction of the diaphragm, should push your fingers out of your lower abdomen. The abdomen is pushing out because the diaphragm is pushing the abdominal contents down (inferiorly); you are feeling the resulting expansion of the abdominal wall.

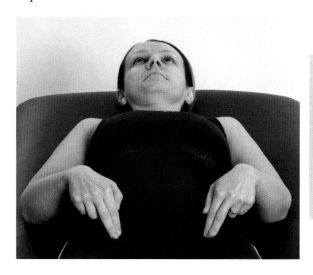

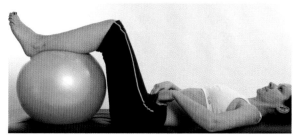

Figure 3.26: During abdominal breathing, there should be an expansion of the abdomen in all three dimensions. You should be able to feel the expansion with your fingers being pushed out of your lower abdominal wall during inspiration.

If your fingers are not being pushed out of your abdominal wall, there are some things that may be inhibiting optimal movement of the diaphragm.

Common causes include:

• Stiffness and/or shortness in the abdominal wall, limiting anterior expansion
• Lack of tonic strength secondary to the spine being chronically locked in thoracolumbar extension (this restricts the diaphragm in an inspiratory position and inhibits it from descending inferiorly during inspiration)
• Excessive upper-chest and neck breathing
• Abdominal fascia or visceral (organ) adhesions or scar tissue formation from previous abdominal or pelvic surgery (cesarean section, hysterectomy, cystectomy, etc.)

Pilates Exercises
We have found Round Back Variations, Knee Stretch Variations, and Elephant are some of the many Pilates exercises that offer good opportunities for teaching and enhancing abdominal breathing patterns. See the exercise section in Chapter 6 for descriptions and photographs of these, and other exercises.

While we have been taught that abdominal breathing (also commonly referred to as *belly breathing*) is ideal, it is only one component of proper breathing. It is somewhat better than using a chest-dominant breathing strategy; however, it is not what we are ultimately striving for. Therefore we will move on to the next component of developing an optimal breathing strategy that is three-dimensional breathing, namely costal, or lateral, breathing.

Costal, or Lateral, Breathing
Costal, or *lateral*, *breathing* refers to the ability to obtain lateral, or side-to-side, expansion of the ribcage. As the diaphragm contracts against its central tendon, it pushes out laterally into the ribcage. Think of this as the opening of an umbrella: as you push up on the central component, the circumference of the umbrella is increased. Similarly, contraction

of the diaphragm, aided by contraction of the intercostal muscles, helps to increase the three-dimensional volume of the ribcage.

To encourage costal breathing, place your hands flat on the lateral aspects of your own or your client's ribcage, just below the chest (Figure 3.27). Take a deep breath in and send the breath laterally into your hands as if you were blowing up a balloon. To facilitate lateral–costal expansion when the thorax is myofascially compressed or stiff, it is helpful to lightly compress the ribcage until about halfway through the inspiratory phase, and then relax the gentle compression through the second half of the inspiration.

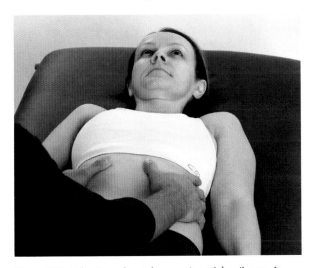

Figure 3.27: Palpation of costal expansion of the ribcage. In individuals with an elevated and stiff anterior ribcage, you can gently traction the anterior aspect of the ribcage inferiorly, or towards the feet, to enhance expiration.

It is common for lateral expansion of the ribcage to be limited, especially in individuals with a stiff thorax that is stuck in an elevated or inspiratory position (Figure 3.28). Lateral costal expansion can be benefited by gently tractioning downward and inward on the ribcage during the expiratory phase of the breath cycle, and holding it lightly to inhibit excessive elevation during the inspiratory phase (see Figure 3.27). This traction should be light and non-painful. You are essentially

trying to facilitate expiration, which is the inferior or downward motion of the thorax as the diaphragm ascends.

Downward traction on the ribcage should not cause change in the neck or upper thorax position and should never be uncomfortable. It should actually create a lengthening in the posterior neck, making it easier to access the deep neck flexors. Additionally, it should help restore more optimal alignment of the thorax relative to the pelvis, thereby enhancing activation of the abdominal wall and pelvic floor.

Place your hands lightly on the lower, lateral aspect of your ribcage. As you breathe out, gently pull your ribcage down towards your feet and towards the midline in an inferior tractioning type of maneuver. This should be a light maneuver, as you are trying to position the ribcage in a position that encourages the diaphragm and other respiratory muscles to facilitate a reflexive inspiratory reaction without tensing other muscles that may inhibit this reaction.

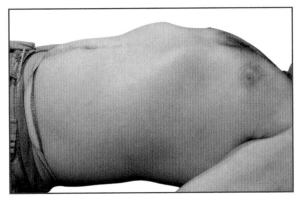

Figure 3.28: A client stuck in an inspiratory position of the ribcage (note the prominence of the lower, anterior aspect of the ribcage).

Several factors can contribute to an inability to get the ribcage to expand laterally, including:

- Hypertonicity of the abdominals, especially the obliques/intercostals and/or erector spinae muscles
- Scar tissue and joint stiffness following thoracic (open heart) or abdominal surgery
- Ribcage stuck in an inspiratory position, contributing to lack of tonic strength in the diaphragm

Improving thoracic mobility is key to correcting many faulty movement patterns, not only those linked to respiration; the low back, hips, shoulders, and neck can also unwittingly be victims of a stiff thoracic spine. This is another reason why it is essential to incorporate a three-dimensional breathing pattern every day.

Some exercises for improving thoracic mobility are given next.

Soft Tissue Release with Balls or a Foam Roller

This procedure can help release abdominal and erector spinae myofascial restrictions. Several different balls of all sizes and densities are available, and each type offers different benefits: larger, softer balls are better for overall mobilizations, while smaller, denser balls can be great for releasing tight erector spinae muscles. Experiment slowly and trust your sensations. We recommend consulting a book on trigger point self-care.

For a broader effect, experiment with placing a soft melon-sized ball between the shoulder blades while lying on your back with knees bent and feet flat. Explore "massaging" this area by bending the spine from side to side. Also try extending your head and shoulders backward over the ball, lengthening the spine as you do so, and then curl up into a crunch, using the abdominals to lift the head

and shoulders (while stabilizing the pelvis in neutral). Alternate these movements several times.

Rolling with a foam roller placed perpendicular to the spine can be another effective way to improve mobility in this area (Figure 3.29). With knees bent and feet flat, roll the spine from the shoulders to the lower ribs (be cautious when rolling over the floating ribs, as they are more delicate). You may want to support your head with your hands to prevent the neck muscles from overworking.

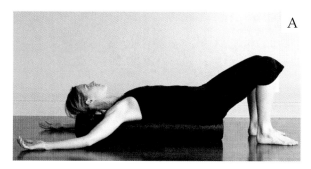

A

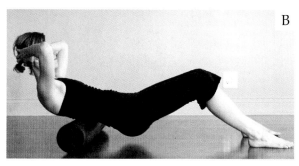

B

Figure 3.29: Foam rolling: (a) along the spine; (b) across the spine.

Rotational Patterns

Several Pilates exercises feature rotational patterns. They offer a fertile opportunity to teach the following important principles of thoracic mobilization:

- Stabilization of the lumbar spine
- Axial elongation to decompress the spine
- Resisting shifting or shearing forces of the vertebrae (and ribs) during rotation
- Lateroposterior breathing to align the pelvic

and respiratory diaphragms and help stabilize the thoracolumbar junction (see later section)

• Mindful attention to spinal articulation in order to improve proprioception, function, agility, and control

Start with the basic patterns and then introduce additional challenges; some examples are given here. See the corrective exercise section in Chapter 6 for more details.

Short Box exercises offer some of the best thoracic mobilization opportunities (e.g., side bends, twists, twists with reach, row the boat). For added proprioceptive challenge, many of these can also be done in a kneeling or standing lunge. Lateral flexion, rotation, flexion, isolated hip hinging, and rolling-up patterns are never boring if you are doing them with the right mindset. Pay close attention to the principles identified above and these exercises will come alive with sensation and challenge. Be creative in the movements. For some Short Box variations inspired by fascial fitness, see the exercise section in Chapter 6.

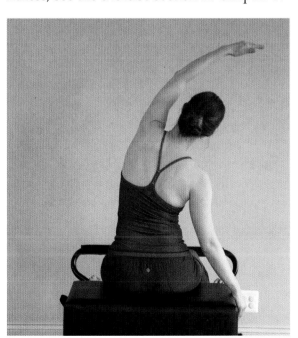

Figure 3.30: Short Box example.

This same sense of fun and exploration can be brought to other thoracic mobilization exercises, such as **Mermaid**. On a hard floor, use a furniture slider (with both hands) to "scrub the floor." Move with a combination of fluidity and gentle bouncing; stretch and articulate the spine in a way that feels good. Move to the front and sides, breathing and working through the areas that feel stuck.

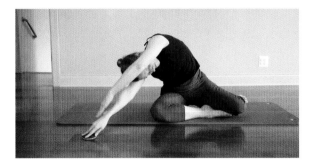

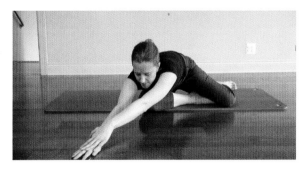

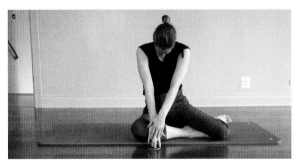

Figure 3.31 : Mermaid variations.

You can also have fun with **quadruped** exercises, such as the ubiquitous Cat/ Cow Stretch, or the **Low Lunge Variations** described here and (with more images) in the exercise section in Chapter 6:

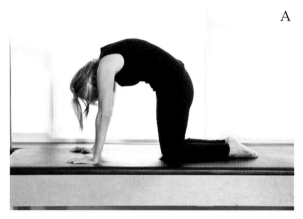

A

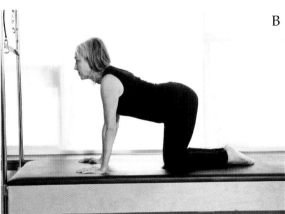

B

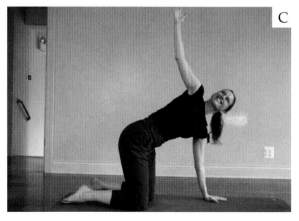

C

Figure 3.32 : Quadruped exercise examples: (a) cat stretch, (b) cow stretch, (c) low lunge.

• Cat/Cow: Rather than just flexing and extending the entire back in an alternating pattern, work to enhance your brain's mental map of your spine by aiming to articulate one vertebra at a time. If you are in a Cat Stretch, begin by curling your tailbone up to the ceiling and then work your way through each segment of your spine, lastly lifting the neck and then the head. To return to a Cat Stretch, begin again at the tailbone, curling it between the legs, and articulating the backbones slowly, working towards the head.

• Practice forward flexion and rotation patterns on all fours (or for more of a challenge, bring one foot forward into a quadruped lunge). Lift one hand and reach it across the midline of the body. With tiny, gentle bounces aimed at the deep rotators of the spine, reach and explore the area between your opposite hand and knee (or hip, if you have stepped your foot forward). Do not stop there. Continue this pulsing reach in the area parallel to the floor above your head and towards your supporting arm.

• Practice thoracic extension and rotation patterns in the quadruped position by rotating one arm away from the midline of the body, towards the ceiling, and then back to the quadruped position. Practice lateral flexion by rotating away from the midline and then reaching the arm parallel to the floor like a Side-Angle Pose in yoga. Finally, the most complex pattern: combine the previous two motions (rotation and lateral flexion) into a freestyle swimming pattern. Ensure that the arm motion begins with thoracic rotation, as this spares the shoulder joint from excess motion and wear and tear.

Posterolateral Breathing

For facilitating proper breathing, the final area we want to focus on is the posterolateral region, where the lower ribs and thoracic spine join the upper region of the lumbar spine. Not only is this region vitally important to the function of the diaphragm, but also the full utilization of a posterolateral breathing strategy enables us to develop optimal intra-abdominal pressure and therefore core stabilization.

This is also an important area, as it is the myofascial intersection of several key stabilizers of the thoracolumbar junction: diaphragm (posterior aspect), psoas, transversus abdominis, and quadratus lumborum. Each of these muscles fascially blends into the thoracolumbar fascia to support the TPC (Figure 3.33). An optimal three-dimensional breathing strategy encourages participation of all these muscles in stabilizing the TPC during functional activity.

imagining blowing up a balloon. If there is correct activity of the diaphragm, when palpating into the posterolateral aspect of the abdominal wall region between the iliac crest and the 12th rib, your fingers should be pushed out of this space as you breathe in (Figures 3.34–35).

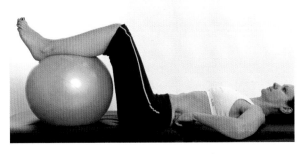

Figure 3.34: Palpation of posterolateral costal expansion.

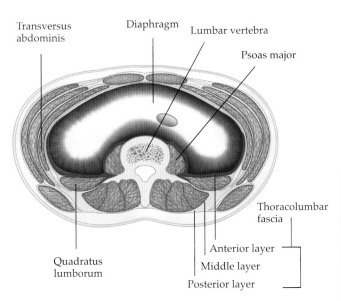

Figure 3.33: The thoracolumbar junction is the region where the diaphragm, psoas, transversus abdominis, and quadratus lumborum blend into the thoracolumbar fascia. Synergistic activation of these muscles, coordinated with three-dimensional breathing, creates the stability required for efficient postural and movement strategies.

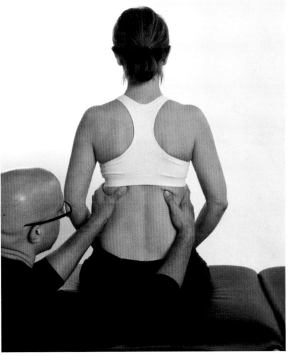

Figure 3.35: Palpation for posterolateral costal expansion as the individual breathes in the upright position. You should note the same expansion whether the individual is lying down or sitting upright.

To encourage posterolateral breathing, place your hands flat on the lateral aspects of the ribcage below the chest and become aware of your posterior ribcage against the surface. Take a deep breath into this region of the ribcage, similarly to earlier when you were

To facilitate posterolateral costal expansion, if the thorax is myofascially compressed or stiff it is helpful to maintain anterior compression over the ribcage as you focus on breathing into the back. As in the case of the stiff thorax that is stuck in an inspiratory position, you can gently traction down and into the ribcage during the expiratory phase of the breath cycle and restrict its motion, to inhibit excessive elevation during the inspiratory cycle.

Several factors can contribute to the inability to get the ribcage to expand posterolaterally, including:

• Increased thoracolumbar extension secondary to faulty stabilization and postural strategies
• Hypertonicity of the lateral division of the oblique abdominals, posterior intercostals, serratus posterior inferior, quadratus lumborum, and/or erector spinae muscles
• The ribcage being stuck in an inspiratory position, contributing to a lack of tonic strength in the diaphragm and transversus abdominis and overstretching of the anterior abdominal wall

Note the thoracolumbar junction extension and increased thoracolumbar erector spinae hypertonicity in the patient with low back pain in Figure 3.36. This is a non-optimal, albeit common, core stabilization strategy that inhibits posterior diaphragm activity and proper function of the entire core system. This strategy also increases compressive forces on the low back and overstretches the anterior abdominals, making it impossible to develop the control required to stabilize the TPC. Thus it is imperative to release the myofascial tone, improve posterolateral expansion during breathing, and then follow up with the proper postural and movement cues to restore a more ideal strategy.

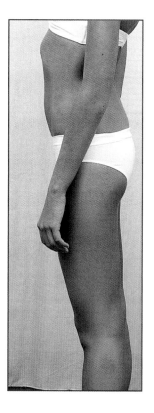

Figure 3.36: Thoracolumbar junction extension and anterior rib cage flare in patient with low back pain.

Some exercises that encourage posterolateral expansion will be discussed next. Pilates exercises—such as Mermaid, Short Box, Round Back, Knee Stretches, and Elephant (see Chapter 6)—provide an excellent opportunity to train posterolateral expansion in the ribcage. As an instructor, placing your hands on the low back and side ribs can be tremendously helpful for a client who is having trouble mentally connecting to this area. Try focusing on expanding the breath into this area during different postures and movements:

• Upright standing or seated (with arms by the sides, then raised in front, then above the head)
• Rotation
• Prone, folded forward over the legs, or in the yoga resting pose known as *Child's Pose*
• Lateral flexion (as in Mermaid)

Training posterolateral expansion (and thoracolumbar stability under load) in supine is an essential part of any Pilates training program. Coaxing clients away from breathing habits that facilitate an unstable TL junction—with lack of integration in the front ribs, and a constricted posterior diaphragm—requires an added level of patience and skill, but there is no reason why even a full room of mat Pilates students cannot learn to recognize and correct this alignment in themselves.

Leg Slides

Begin with feet flat, knees bent, and hands on the stomach. This is the easiest position for learning to expand the posterolateral ribs. From the supine, bent-knee, neutral-pelvis position:

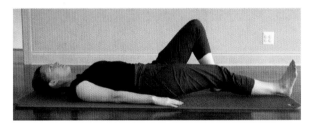

Figure 3.37: Leg slides.

1. Breathe in, feeling the fullness in the low back ribs. Breathe out, feeling the front ribs integrating. Continue to breathe in this way, maintaining the low back rib contact with the mat for the entire breath cycle.

2. Keeping this contact, slide one leg long down the mat. If the ribs start to pop, pause and return the leg to the start position. Alternate legs in this way.

3. Now try this with just the arms. One arm reaches up to the ceiling and falls backward towards the floor. If the ribs pop, pause and return to the start position. Alternate arm reaches in this way.

4. Finally, slide one leg and reach the opposite arm backward, maintaining lower-rib contact with the mat the entire time. Alternate sides.

Note

If the shoulders are tight, they will try to "borrow" extra range by lifting up on the front ribs when the arms reach back. This movement of popping the front ribs works against core stability.

By the same token, if the core is weak and/or the low back and hip flexors are tight, then sliding the legs long and straight down the mat will also cause the ribs to pop up. This is a situation of the tail wagging the dog. Learn to make an anchor of neutral pelvis and neutral ribcage so that all muscles may come into their natural balance.

Marching Steps and Lower Lifts

From Leg Slides, we can progress to Marching Steps, and finally to Lower Lifts (with extended knees).

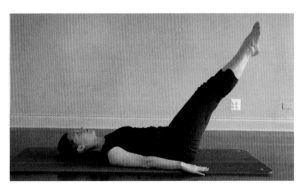

Figure 3.38: Marching steps and lower lifts.

1. First progression: Begin in the supine, bent-knee, neutral-pelvis position. Lift one knee up above the hip, maintaining lower-rib contact with the mat. Return to the mat and alternate sides.

2. Second progression: Begin in table top position (feet lifted off the floor, knees above the hips). Drop one foot to the floor, maintaining a 90-degree angle at the knee and lower-rib contact with the mat. Raise the foot back to the start position. Alternate sides.

3. Third progression: Lower Lift (modified variation). Both knees lower any amount towards the floor, maintaining lower-rib contact with the mat and front rib integration. Be sure that the pelvis remains stable so as not to strain the low back. Lift back to the start position and repeat. In variations 3 and 4, inhale as the legs move away, and exhale as they move toward, the body.

4. Fourth progression: Lower Lift (full variation). Both legs are fully extended and lower together any amount towards the floor, maintaining lower-rib contact with the mat and front rib integration. Be sure that the pelvis remains stable so as not to strain the low back. Lift back to the start position and repeat.

Bridging

On the reformer: lower the headrest and attach two to five springs (start heavier and reduce tension to increase the challenge).

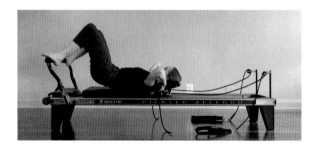

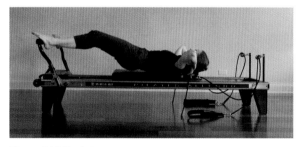

Figure 3.39: Bridging.

1. Lying on your back, place the heels of the feet wide on the footbar. (Footbar on the top setting.)

2. Roll up (starting with the hips) to the lowest ribs. In other words, the lowest ribs should be touching the mat, but the hips should be lifted.

3. Breathe into this band across the low back ribs (the thoracolumbar junction) and feel the ribs expand into the mat. Softly thread the front ribs together, as if you were tying a corset.

4. Press through the feet and extend the legs, moving the carriage away from the footbar, breathing naturally. Try not to allow the low back ribs to lose contact with the mat.

5. Return the carriage to the start position, maintaining the position of the spine (hips lifted and low back ribs touching the mat).

6. Continue this movement, in and out, concentrating on breathing into the low back ribs and threading the front ribs.

On the mat: lie supine, with feet flat and knees bent. Much like on the reformer, roll up until you can feel the bottom of the ribcage pressing into the mat. If your low back is tight or the back of the legs are weak, you may have more success initially by resting the sacrum on a yoga block. Hold this posture and breathe into the band across the low back ribs. For an added challenge, try lifting one leg and then the other, while continuing to feel the low back ribs expanding into the mat.

Wall Angels

This exercise is easy for clients to practice at home and offers a number of benefits, from shoulder opening and strengthening to spinal elongation and improving breathing habits. When the TPC is in ideal alignment (i.e., respiratory and pelvic diaphragms are parallel), the low back ribs are in contact with the wall and there is a small lumbar curve. The added extension at the arms and shoulders provides an additional challenge, as tight pectoral muscles will "borrow" from the neutral alignment of the spine, pulling the ribcage forward, off the wall. In the beginning, establish neutral spine and promote the proprioceptive feedback afforded by the wall as the client learns to breath into the low back ribs. Allow the arms to be off the wall until adequate length is eventually achieved in the anterior shoulder muscles. Move the arms up and down ten times, breathing into the back and elongating the neck and spine.

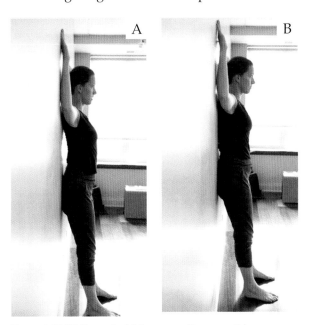

Figure 3.39: Wall angels, (a) Incorrect alignment. (b) Correct alignment.

Whether in a prone, upright, supine, or other position, it is essential to train these thoracic stabilization patterns with the appropriate amount of load. Starting with minimal load before advancing to more challenging variations (e.g., starting with Marching Steps before progressing to Lower Lifts, and mastering quadruped patterns before advancing to Plank variations) will ensure that your body and brain are integrating these patterns and that you have the requisite strength to take on more.

Rate and Frequency of Optimal Breathing

While there are various recommendations regarding the optimal number of breaths per minute an individual should take and how long each phase of the breath cycle should last, we generally use the following guidelines:

• Ideally, there should be approximately 8–12 breaths per minute
• The expiration should last approximately twice as long as the inspiration; this facilitates optimal emptying of the lungs and sets up the necessary neural-driven reflexes for facilitating the corresponding inhalation
• There should be about a 1-second pause between the inspiratory and expiratory phases; this pause serves to slow down the rate of breathing and reduces the likelihood of hyperventilation, which commonly occurs during breath retraining

In practice, the breathing pattern would be as follows:

• Breathe in for 4 seconds (count one one-thousand, two one-thousand, three one-thousand, four one-thousand)
• Pause for 1 second (one one-thousand)
• Breathe out for 7 seconds (one one-thousand, two one-thousand, etc. up to 7 seconds)
• Pause for 1 second (one one-thousand)
• Repeat the cycle

People with significant respiratory dysfunction might perform only one or two cycles of this breathing pattern before returning to their regular breathing strategy. For those with a more optimal strategy, perform two to five cycles before returning to quiet, resting respiratory patterns. As clients progress and their myofascial and pulmonary systems adapt, work towards three to five sets of three to five breaths in this manner. The important determinant of how many sets and repetitions you ultimately do is based on optimal completion of the pattern without compensation. And of course, the ultimate goal is to have this breathing strategy become a habitual method of breathing in daily life.

Additional Benefits of Developing Optimal Respiratory Patterns

Along with oxygenation and stabilization, establishing three-dimensional respiration provides three additional benefits that deserve mention because they directly relate to our spinal health and overall health in general.

1. **Mobilization of the trunk and spine.** As the diaphragm contracts and pulls against its attachments along the trunk and spine, it gently mobilizes the spine. Motion of the diaphragm, because it also has attachments around the thorax, facilitates mobility of the entire trunk and spine. In this manner, three-dimensional breathing facilitates trunk and spine mobility, and trunk and spine mobility in turn facilitates three-dimensional breathing.

2. **Massage of the viscera.** Mobility and blood flow to the organs is critical to a healthy visceral system (Wetzler 2014). The diaphragm sits directly on top of the abdominal viscera and directly below the lungs and heart. When the diaphragm contracts, it pushes inferiorly into the abdominal contents while creating space above for the lungs and heart. Mobility of the diaphragm quite literally massages and mobilizes the viscera while facilitating the flow of blood and lymph through the abdominal and pelvic regions.

3. **Management of emotions.** Optimal respiration is one of the most effective ways to bring awareness and focus to a task and aids greatly in managing emotional stress. Performing deep, diaphragmatic or three-

dimensional breathing can quickly switch our body from a strategy that is sympathetic nervous system dominant (common when we are stressed, anxious, or frustrated and characterized by shallow, rapid breathing) to one that is parasympathetic nervous system dominant, which is more conducive to rest and regeneration of the body (Osar 2012, Umphred 2007).

Step 3—Coordination

For some clients, simply improving their three-dimensional breathing strategy is enough to improve recruitment and activation of the deep myofascial system (diaphragm, transversus abdominis, psoas, pelvic floor, quadratus lumborum, multifidi). However, in the case of muscle inhibition (especially if it has been a long-term issue or there has been abdominal, pelvic, thoracic, or lumbar surgery), specific activation techniques are required to activate or "turn on" the deep myofascial system.

Deep myofascial activation must be coordinated with respiration, because the activity of this deep system provides the segmental joint stabilization required to resist the pull or contraction of the superficial movement system. In this synergistic capacity, the diaphragm and abdominals, along with the rest of the deep myofascial system, stabilize the TPC. This coordinated function is compromised most when there is injury, trauma, surgery, inflammation, or some other stressor that inhibits either proper respiration or optimal activation of the deep myofascial system. True core stability, then, is the ability to coordinate activation of the deep myofascial system with three-dimensional breathing and sustain this synergy throughout any functional activity or Pilates exercise.

Coordinate and Maintain

True core stability is the ability to coordinate optimal respiration with activation of the deep myofascial system and maintain this synergistic activity throughout functional activities.

Coordination of Breathing and Core Activation

We will refer to the strategy of coordinating activation of the deep myofascial system with diaphragmatic breathing as the *Breath Activation Strategy* (BAS). The BAS is not just a simple action of bracing or co-activating all the muscles around the core to create stability. The central component of the BAS is that we pre-activate or preferentially recruit the deep myofascial system and are able to sustain this activation as we breathe, with little or no contribution from the superficial myofascial system unless it is required for a particular activity.

This is important as it gives us an opportunity to activate and build endurance using a low-level strategy as opposed to being restricted to only using a high-level "bracing" type of strategy. This provides us with the stability required for joint control and simultaneously develops an optimal and non-compensatory strategy for low-level tasks, such as sitting, standing, bending, walking, and rotating.

As mentioned previously, when we have core dysfunction secondary to muscle inhibition, our nervous system generally defaults to using a high-level or bracing stabilization strategy for most of our activities. In the long term this not only affects our ability to breathe three-dimensionally and generate optimal levels of IAP, but also increases compressive demands on the joints, which in turn becomes a major contributor to soft tissue injuries and degenerative joint disease.

Incorporate the Breath Activation Strategy

The BAS enables us to develop a low-level stabilization strategy that is important for activating and building endurance of the deep myofascial system and for coordinating this activity with three-dimensional breathing. This is one of the most important steps in developing a well-balanced and efficient core stabilization strategy.

The BAS is specifically designed to improve motor control rather than strength. Motor control is the ability to coordinate the timing, intensity, and endurance of muscle activation and ensures that it is appropriate for the task in hand. Motor control also ensures that muscles are firing when and how they should in order to create optimal stability and movement.

Strengthening should only occur once motor control has been restored, otherwise we are just strengthening a dysfunctional strategy. Strengthening on top of poor motor control can be likened to developing a faulty golf swing and then playing year after year, thereby "strengthening" the faulty neural patterns that have been created. Instead, you could invest your time in learning the nuances of a more optimal swing pattern (coordination, timing, and control) and focus on integrating this into your current golf game. Generally, you struggle more at the beginning, but in the long term, you are learning the proper neurological patterns that will enhance your golf game.

Pilates patterns to improve core strength will be developed in Chapter 6; these are used once the individual has developed a more efficient strategy of motor control.

Coordinate Muscle Activity

Motor control is the nervous system coordination of timing, intensity, and endurance of muscle activity to ensure that the myofascial system is working as it should in order to create optimal stability and movement. Strengthening should only occur once motor control has been restored.

The BAS begins with activation of the anterior aspect of the TVA, as this is the easiest area for most individuals to become aware of and 'feel' muscle recruitment. Once activation can be felt in the anterior portion, we will also want to ensure that the lateral and posterior aspects are involved. Additionally, activating the anterior aspect of the TVA will enhance the ability to activate the lateral and posterior aspects, which are generally more challenging.

Assuming that you have an optimal respiratory strategy, place your hands inside your ASISs. Take a deep breath in and let all the air out; now hold your breath out. Create light tension in your lower abdominal wall— essentially the TVA—by trying not to let your fingers get pushed further into the abdominal wall.

You should note a slight tensioning underneath your fingers to ensure that you are activating the transversus abdominis and not the obliques. Any aggressive tensioning, drawing in, or activation will result in activation of the internal or external oblique, and will bypass the ability to use the TVA to enhance segmental stability of the spine, pelvis, and trunk. You should feel a very light tension, almost as if a layer of plastic wrap is being tensed under your fingers. If your fingers are being pushed out of the abdominal region, this is a substitution from the abdominal obliques and usually occurs as the individual wants to make this activation "harder" or "firmer"; more is not better when trying to restore activation of

the deep myofascial system. Less truly is more when we are attempting to activate the deep myofascial system.

Once you have this myofascial activation, take a three-dimensional breath in and out while maintaining the activation. As you exhale fully, lightly hold your breath and see if you can feel the relaxation of the TVA to ensure that you have maintained coordination of muscle activation and respiration. Repeat this strategy as many times as you can. Initially it will be challenging, but with time the process will get easier, and you will be able to perform it is effortlessly with your three-dimensional breathing.

Once you have activated the anterior portion of the abdominal wall, you must be able to activate the posterolateral portion of the TVA—the fibers that wrap around the body between the ribcage and top of the iliac crest and insert into the thoracolumbar fascia. Place your fingers between your lowest rib and your iliac crest as you did when you were attempting to breathe posterolaterally. Now perform the same sequence as above to activate the anterior portion of the muscle. Take a deep breath in and let it all out. Holding it out, create that light tension by resisting your fingers pushing into your lateral abdomen. Maintain this activation as you take a deep breath in and out. Hold your breath out and ensure that you have maintained the activation during your breathing.

Another strategy used by many physical therapists and pelvic floor specialists is to activate the pelvic floor, which should co-activate with the TVA. Preferential activation of the pelvic floor can be effective for achieving co-contraction of the TVA. These cues can be especially helpful for individuals experiencing urinary incontinence following childbirth, hysterectomies, or prostate surgery. The pelvic floor (urogenital diaphragm) needs to resist the activity of the diaphragm, and when inhibited by poor respiratory habits, trauma, and/or surgery, it needs to be activated in a similar way to the TVA.

There are several effective strategies for obtaining activation of the pelvic floor:

• Visualize gently lifting the anus, vagina (in females), or testicles (in males)
• Create an image of a tension wire connecting your tailbone to the back of your pubic bone
• Imagine a hammock or elevator floor between your tailbone and pubic bone that is gently lifting the region up

Regardless of the cue used, when retraining activation of the TVA and pelvic floor, there should be no change in the alignment of the pelvis or lumbar spine and no change in the ability to maintain three-dimensional breathing. Change in alignment, over-gripping the glutes or hip rotators, and holding the breath are considered non-optimal activation strategies and will perpetuate poor stabilization stereotypes.

Rate and Frequency of Optimal Coordination

The initial motor control training we have been developing is designed to restore optimal coordination between respiration and activation. The goal is to maintain activation of the deep myofascial system for one to three breath cycles. Once an optimal strategy is developed, the emphasis shifts to building up endurance, which can be accomplished by increasing the number of sets and repetitions. Initially the individual works up to performing five sets of five deep breaths per set, and then to the point where they are essentially able to maintain the coordination for the duration of their exercise pattern. Ultimately, BAS training is designed to help you develop your

subconscious strategy for stabilization, both during your session and during activities of daily life (Figure 3.40).

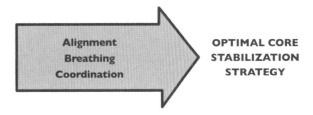

Figure 3.40: The development of an optimal core stabilization strategy derives from the ability to align the diaphragms (the fascial covering at the top of the lungs, the respiratory diaphragm, and the urogenital diaphragm), perform three-dimensional breathing, and coordinate respiration with activation of the deep myofascial system. When we develop an optimal core stabilization strategy, we can maintain our posture and move with greater ease, and there is less likelihood of developing the compensatory strategies that lead to tightness, dysfunction, and eventually pain.

Achieve Core Stability
True core stability is achieved when one can coordinate three-dimensional breathing with activation of the deep abdominal wall and maintain this strategy through functional Pilates exercises or activities of daily life.

Dysfunction of the Breath Activation Strategy
Understanding optimal respiratory mechanics and how they relate to developing an efficient core stabilization strategy is essential when designing and implementing a Pilates program. However, it is equally important to recognize the signs of non-optimal respiratory mechanics. As we have briefly discussed throughout this chapter, non-optimal respiratory mechanics results in faulty stabilization of the core. Faulty stabilization then requires the overuse of certain muscles and leads to muscle imbalances, which distort posture and in turn lead to greater compensations.

For example, one common dysfunction we briefly discussed earlier that leads to many individuals being unable to perform ideal three-dimensional breathing (and therefore stabilize their core) is not being able to achieve a full expiration. These individuals often present with a wide, flared ribcage and prominent lower ribs (Figure 3.41). They will generally be good belly breathers and yet be unable to bring the anterior portion of the ribcage down during expiration. They will also likely struggle to breathe posterolaterally as they are usually locked into thoracolumbar hyperextension.

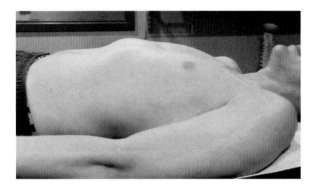

Figure 3.41: This individual is unable to achieve a full expiration—notice the wide, flared ribcage and prominent lower ribs.

Not being able to achieve a full expiration or return to a more neutral position of the thorax during the respiratory cycle presents several challenges to developing optimal respiration and intra-abdominal pressure:

• It inhibits the reflexive action of the primary respiratory muscles that should facilitate the next breath. Therefore, the individual has to overuse their accessory muscles to help them breathe more fully, which leads to increased hypertonicity in these muscles and perpetuates forward-head and forward-shoulder postures and faulty respiratory mechanics

• When diaphragm motion is limited by a stiff thorax and is not able to descend to its optimal resting alignment, its contribution to respiration is diminished, requiring compensatory overuse of the accessory muscles

• The lack of optimal thorax movement does not allow the diaphragm to move through its normal patterns; the diaphragm is therefore unable to contribute to overall thoracic and spinal mobility. This perpetuates the cycle of thoracic stiffness, diaphragm hypomobility, and overuse of the accessory muscles of respiration

The inability to balance the deep and superficial myofascial systems and generate IAP through three-dimensional breathing, while perhaps not a major problem in the short term, gradually leads to dramatic changes within the system. Over time, the effects of being unable to utilize an efficient BAS can be quite devastating to overall function.

Recall our previous analogy of the box full of eggs internally supported by a stability ball. Imagine you took the plug out of the stability ball so that the air escapes. What happens now when you sit on the box of eggs? The ball and box collapse and you crush the eggs. This is similar to what happens over time when we do not optimally breathe, co-activate the deep myofascial system, and generate the intra-abdominal pressure required to stabilize the trunk and spine. The forces of gravity, external loads, our own body weight, and overuse of a compensatory high-level strategy will progressively virtually compress the spine.

There are three primary issues associated with the inability to optimally use the BAS:

1. It is one of the leading contributors to degenerative disc disease, as prolonged disc compression leads to disc degeneration. Disc degeneration eventually leads to narrowing of the spinal canal, where the spinal cord is located, as well as of the foraminal canal, which is where the peripheral nerves exit the spine to travel through the body. Over-compression of the spine is a leading cause of degenerative disc disease and spinal stenosis (narrowing of the spinal canal) as we age.

2. It also contributes to degenerative joint disease, more commonly referred to as *osteoarthritis*. It is simply Wolff's law in action: increased stress on a bone or joint will increase bone production, hence the growth of bone spurs and thickening of the joints around the spine when there is an inability to generate IAP to decompress the system. Along with disc degeneration, this bony growth can decrease the size of either the spinal or foraminal canal, compressing soft tissue structures, such as nerves and ligaments.

Additionally, this non-optimal stabilization strategy creates hypertrophy or thickening of the tissues surrounding the spine, such as the ligaments and joint capsules. Thickening of the ligamentum flavum (the ligament that supports the lamina or posterior aspect of the vertebrae) is another significant contributor to spinal stenosis as well as back pain as we age.

3. With an ideal BAS we are able to balance out the contraction of the superficial myofascial system and reduce stress and pressure upon our joints. IAP is an important strategy for controlling internal pressure; however, when there is over-contraction or increased use of the superficial myofascial system for stabilization, there is increased pressure placed on the lower abdomen and pelvis. Without an ideal BAS to develop IAP, external pressure and internal stresses begin to push out into the lower abdomen and down into the pelvic floor. It has been surmised that this lack of pressure control is a likely contributor to diastasis recti in active individuals, lower abdominal distension, sports hernias, and incontinence (Osar 2014).

The Psoas

The psoas deserves a special mention because of its important contributions to core stability and its implications for low back and hip dysfunction. While not meant to be comprehensive, this section will provide insight into this often-misunderstood muscle. The psoas (Figure 3.42) has proximal attachments to the anterior surface—both the transverse processes and vertebral bodies—of vertebral levels T12–L5. It also has attachments directly into the anterior aspects of the intervertebral discs themselves. Distally it crosses the anterior aspect of the pelvis to attach into the lesser trochanter of the femur.

If we looked simply at its origin and insertion, it would seem that the psoas was well suited to hip flexion. However, one question that should be asked if we are to believe that the psoas is truly a primary hip flexor is: why does it attach to every level of the lumbar spine and even extend up into the lower thoracic spine? Furthermore, there are two additional important regions of attachments that provide some insight into the functional role of the psoas.

The psoas has proximal fascial attachments into the diaphragm and transversus abdominis, and distally it fascially blends with the pelvic floor (Gibbons 2005). In fact, research has demonstrated that the psoas is primarily a spine stabilizer (Hu et al. 2011). A unilateral straight-leg raise performed in the supine position activates the contralateral or non-moving psoas, suggesting its role in spinal stabilization.

Likely functioning as part of the deep myofascial system, the psoas also helps to maintain centering of the femoral head within the acetabulum (Gibbons 2005).

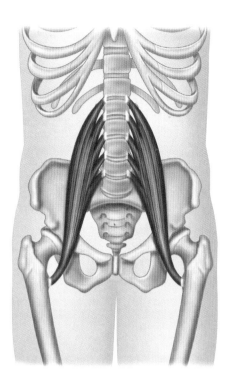

Figure 3.42: The psoas.

Additionally, MRI studies on individuals with low back pain have demonstrated atrophy in both the multifidi and psoas (Barker et al. 2000). Recall that when there is pain and/or inflammation, the muscles of the deep myofascial system seem to be preferentially inhibited.

It appears that it is truly time to rethink the implications of the psoas for low back pain and hip dysfunction and the important role this muscle plays in core stabilization.

Many rehabilitation protocols for anterior pelvic tilt, low back pain, and hip tightness are based on stretching the "tight, short" psoas. In my (Evan's) clinical experience, I rarely find clients' or patients' psoas muscles to be short and tight. In fact, I often find the psoas to be over-lengthened and weak in manual muscle tests in individuals with core and hip dysfunction. This often necessitates the overuse of the superficial erector spinae muscles in the role of spine stabilization, and the superficial hip flexors—primarily the rectus femoris and tensor fasciae latae—in the role of hip flexion. Many patients and clients complain about having tightness in these muscles and it is also where we tend to find significant myofascial hypertonicity and trigger points. These individuals grip from their back and/or anterior hip to aid hip flexion and postural support of the TPC when there is psoas inhibition (Osar 2012, Osar 2014).

Many practitioners blame an anterior pelvic tilt and psoas shortness on the seated posture. In other words, they suggest we sit in an anterior pelvic tilt all day, shortening the muscles to reflect this position once we stand. It is actually quite challenging to sit in an anterior pelvic tilt, unless you consciously attempt to do so. Most of our society tends to sit in a posterior rather than an anterior pelvic tilt (Figure 3.43). It is the posterior pelvic tilt created from sitting and cueing habits—examples include 'pull your abs in' or 'tuck your tailbone under' or 'flatten your low back'—that significantly contributes to psoas inhibition and a resultant loss of core stability and hip control (Osar 2012, Osar 2014).

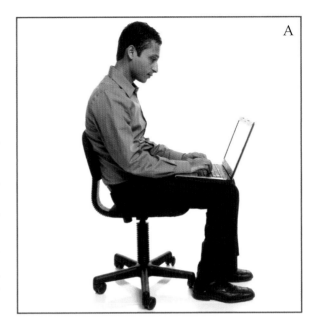

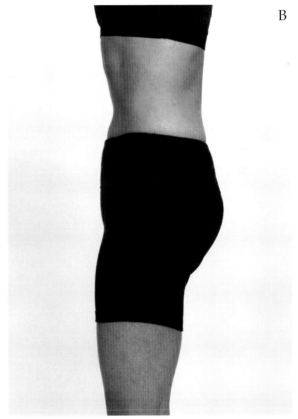

Figure 3.43: (a) An individual sitting with his thorax behind his pelvis and the pelvis posteriorly tilted. This is a common sitting posture that creates inhibition of the psoas and leads to low back and hip dysfunction. (b) Posterior pelvic tilt and flattening of the lumbar spine in a client who has been overly cued to 'pull her abs in' and 'tuck her pelvis under'. This client presented with chronic low back pain and tight hips with associated psoas inhibition.

Evaluating Psoas Length—The Modified Thomas Test

The Modified Thomas Test is the gold standard for evaluating the length of the hip flexors, including the rectus femoris, tensor fasciae latae, and psoas. The test is performed by having the individual sit at the end of the table, pull one thigh into their chest, and lie back to evaluate the hanging leg.

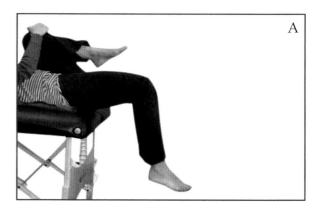

Positive findings in the Thomas Test include:

- If the thigh is held above the level of the table: psoas tightness (Figure 3.44(a))
- If the thigh abducts and the tibia is in external rotation: tensor fasciae latae and iliotibial band tightness (Figure 3.44(b))
- If the angle at the knee is greater than 90 degrees: rectus femoris tightness (Figure 3.44(c))

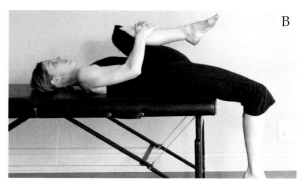

Myofascial tightness of the anterior thigh, however, can create a false positive for psoas tightness in this test. True psoas involvement is when the thigh is above the height of the table *and* you are able to palpate hypertonicity (tautness) in the psoas muscle belly, just inside the inguinal ligament. If the thigh is above the height of the table and no palpable hypertonicity is felt in the psoas, the leg is being held up by myofascial tension in the anterior thigh rather than by a short psoas (Osar 2014).

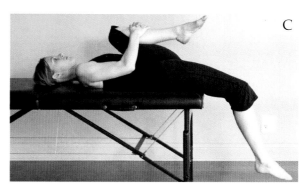

Figure 3.44: Modified Thomas Test: (a) positive test for psoas shortness—the knee is above the height of the table; (b) proper length of the hip flexors—the knee is level with the thigh; (c) over-lengthened psoas—the knee is below the level of the thigh.

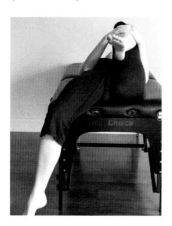

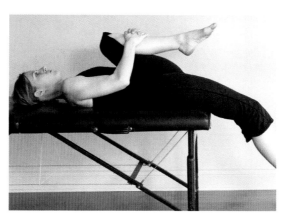

Figure 3.45: Modified Thomas Test: (a) shortness of the tensor fasciae latae and iliotibial band—the leg should be in line with the body rather than abducted; (b) shortness of the rectus femoris—the knee should be flexed at a right angle when at normal length (right).

The patient in Figure 3.46 presented with low back discomfort and hip tightness. Her therapist instructed her to stretch her psoas and perform posterior pelvic tilts as part of her rehabilitation program because she was told that she was in an anterior pelvic tilt and this was what was causing her low back pain. You can see from her Modified Thomas Test that her psoas is actually too long; her leg should be in line with her body, but it is actually lower than her body. This is a common finding in individuals with hip and low back issues. This patient also demonstrates thoracolumbar extension, which is commonly mistaken for an anterior pelvic tilt.

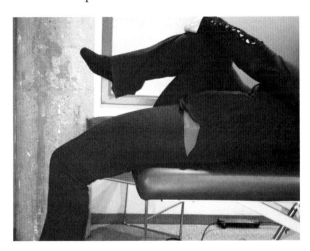

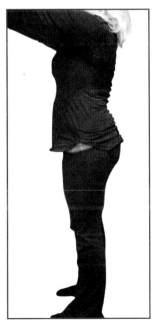

Figure 3.46: Modified Thomas Test results for a patient presenting with low back discomfort and hip tightness.

Activating the Psoas

In individuals with an over-lengthened and inhibited psoas (the psoas is over-lengthened during the Thomas test and tests weak on a manual muscle test), the psoas will be activated similarly to the rest of the deep myofascial system. There should be preferential activation of the deep myofascial system (transversus abdominis, pelvic floor, and psoas, for example) just prior to recruitment of their functional synergists (external obliques, glutes, and iliacus). The goal during retraining is to preferentially activate the psoas without simultaneously engaging the superficial hip flexors (rectus femoris and tensor fasciae latae) or the adductors. Recall that we are attempting to change the timing of the firing between the deep hip muscles and the superficial muscles, rather than suggest that the superficial muscles are not required for hip flexion.

The psoas will be recruited similarly to the deep myofascial system as described earlier. Lying supine with the leg over a stability ball or chair (Figure 3.47), activate your deep myofascial system as you did earlier. Your other hand will palpate the front of your hip to ensure that you are not overly recruiting the rectus femoris, tensor fasciae latae, or adductors. Visualize a deep wire connecting the front of your spine—the origin of the psoas—to the front of your hip near the groin area, where the psoas attaches into the lesser trochanter of the femur. Maintaining the activation of the deep myofascial system that we discussed earlier, slowly slide your leg along the ball or chair (flexing your hip) and return to the start position. Because this is a low-level activation strategy, the superficial hip flexors are not required to participate in this movement and should remain relaxed and soft throughout this pattern. Perform three to five sets of five repetitions and then integrate the psoas into your Pilates patterns, such as heel slides, leg lowering, and Leg Circles.

Anchoring at the psoas origin in the lumbar spine and lifting the hips resembles the developing infant's earliest "psoas exercise" as they grab the toes and place them in their mouth (Figure 3.48). Adding Leg Springs for support (and eliminating the toe-tasting bit!) is an excellent way to practice this primitive movement pattern in the adult body.

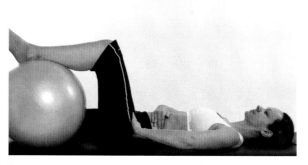

Figure 3.47: Palpating for recruitment of the TVA and psoas during hip flexion. The superficial hip flexors should remain relatively soft and relaxed as the hip is flexed towards the chest.

Special Note to Pilates Instructors

Liz Koch, author of *The Psoas Book* (2012), believes that sitting behind the sitz bones in a posterior tuck of the pelvis can overstretch the ligaments of the sacroiliac joints, creating tension along the spinal midline and resulting in a shortened, overworked psoas. In contrast to this viewpoint, the concept is worth exploring in clients with psoas involvement resulting from true shortness in the muscle. What we, the authors of this book, have in common with her is the recognition that developing a kinesthetic awareness of the psoas (whether short, overstretched, inhibited, or overactive) is key to restoring function and balance to the core.

Additionally, take note of what poet and essayist Ralph Waldo Emerson so famously wrote: "People only see what they are prepared to see." Many of us in the health and fitness field have only been prepared (taught) to see an anterior pelvic tilt and psoas shortness. Be sure to follow up what you find in your postural evaluations with other assessments—such as movement evaluation, range of motion, and/or muscle tests—before you make your exercise recommendations.

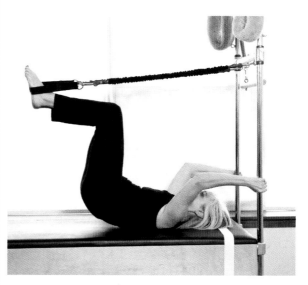

Figure 3.48: Activating the psoas in conjunction with the abdominals using spring support.

Conclusion

The myofascial system is an integral component in developing an efficient core stabilization strategy. By developing three-dimensional breathing and coordinating it with activation of the deep myofascial system we are able to generate the intra-abdominal pressure required to stabilize and decompress our TPC. Through myofascial connections, both the deep and superficial myofascial systems create fascial tension and suspension that stabilize the trunk, spine, and pelvis.

Through a coordinated breathing and activation strategy, the myofascial systems seamlessly contribute to creating optimal levels of joint stability to support posture and movement, while reducing the potentially damaging forces of shear, rotation, and tension that occur during functional activities. Thus optimal core function relies on the delicate balance, coordination, and control of respiration, activation, and integration into functional movement. Imbalance between the myofascial systems and fascial restrictions, as well as developing non-optimal habits in any region of the body, can create dramatic effects on our core stability, which impacts both posture and movement. We will look at the development of non-optimal posture and movement in the next chapter.

Use an Integrative Approach to Achieve Optimal Core Stability
- Three-dimensional breathing develops intra-abdominal pressure, allowing the spine to be long and resistant to compression.
- Activation of the deep myofascial system creates proximal joint control.
- The superficial myofascial system adds just the right amount of joint compression while facilitating movement of the body.

Collectively, these actions contribute to optimal core stabilization and the development of the desired "long and lean"—and controlled—appearance associated with Pilates training.

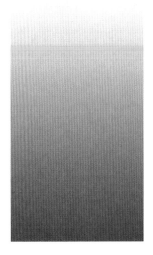

Dysfunction of the Core

4

In Chapter 3 we discussed how the nervous system coordinates the activity of the deep and superficial nervous systems with three-dimensional breathing to create optimal core stabilization. Recall that having an efficient core stabilization strategy is not just about being able to activate solely the transversus abdominis or simply bracing one's core in an attempt to create a rigid TPC; efficiency is about developing a strategy that allows us to maintain proper breathing, protect our joints, and adapt to the demands of life. The more adaptable our core stabilization strategy is, the more efficient our body will be in performing the tasks that we need and want to do on a regular basis.

We demonstrated in the previous chapter an approach for developing efficient core stabilization so that we are able to use the appropriate stabilization strategy for the posture and movement required for low-level tasks—such as walking, sitting, and standing—and tasks that require increased levels of stability—such as lifting a heavy box, running, or performing a side Plank pattern during a Pilates session.

In this chapter we will discuss common reasons why many individuals develop non-optimal core stabilization strategies and how they directly lead to faulty postural and movement patterns. We will specifically look at how inhibition of the deep myofascial system and over-activation of the superficial myofascial system directly impact core function and affect performance in other regions of the body, such as the hips. Finally, we will identify the short- and long-term effects that these non-optimal strategies have on posture and movement.

The benefits of understanding the concepts relating to the development of core dysfunction include:

• It will enable you to identify the three common causes of non-optimal core stabilization and explain how the nervous system compensates for non-optimal core stabilization strategies.
• It will allow you to recognize the common postural and movement dysfunctions that result from non-optimal stabilization strategies, either in yourself or in your clients if you are a Pilates instructor.

• If you are a Pilates instructor, it will help you educate your students about the rationale for developing a more efficient core stabilization strategy rather than simply trying to strengthen the weak, inhibited muscles and stretch the tight, overactive muscles.

There are three primary reasons why we develop non-optimal core stabilization strategies:

• Neurodevelopment: non-optimal neuro-motor patterns acquired through childhood development
• Trauma: acute trauma, repetitive or cumulative trauma from habitual postures and patterns, and/or surgery, which creates scar tissue, muscle inhibition, and compensatory strategies
• Habituation: learned postural and move-ment strategies that perpetuate non-optimal core function

For some, a combination of these three factors contributes to their individual strategy. The important thing is not to become obsessed by the cause(s) that contribute to the development of dysfunctional strategies by individuals, but rather to better understand the reasons behind the development of non-optimal posture and movement. This information helps us then develop a more efficient core stabilization strategy that supports optimal posture and movement.

Neurodevelopment

Each of us is born with an inherent or natural ability to stabilize and move. During proper development of the neuromotor (nervous and muscular) system, there are specific neurally ingrained and predetermined patterns of stabilization that dictate the postural and movement patterns we will use throughout life. In optimal development, the postural stabilization function precedes the development of movement: in other words, we begin learning postural stability prior to being able to carry out purposeful movement.

For example, in the first trimester of life, an infant will begin developing phasic muscle (muscles that tend to be part of the superficial myofascial system) activity and co-activation of muscle antagonists. This coordinated muscle development will help the child develop control of their head and learn how to stabilize in the supine and prone positions (Figure 4.1).

During the second trimester of life, the diaphragm shifts its function from purely respiratory to one that includes postural support as well. The ability of the deep myofascial system to develop and sustain intra-abdominal pressure plays a significant role in early spine development and stabilization. It is also during this time that coordination between the deep and superficial myofascial systems creates joint centration, or the position that best aligns the joint for loading and rotation.

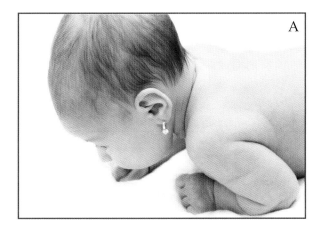

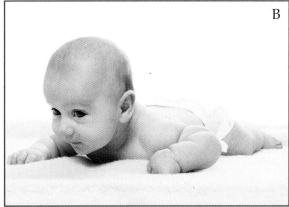

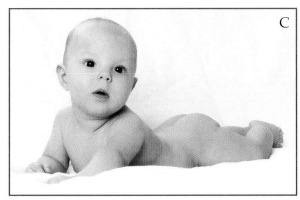

Figure 4.1: Example of prone developmental progression. Prone postural support function develops from the first trimester through the beginning of the second where the child goes from support with the arms just below the height of the shoulders (a), to the level of the shoulders (b), and finally to in front of the shoulders (c). In the last position, the child develops the core stabilization required to push themselves up with support upon their forearms. The prone pattern is important for the ability to elongate the spine during extension, rather than lifting by creating hyperextension at the thoracolumbar junction.

Understanding this early progression can help us develop proper exercise progressions for clients with non-optimal core or shoulder support in the prone position. For example, the prone lengthening position (Figure 4.2) is an excellent pattern using this concept to develop the core and scapular control required for other supine patterns such as Mermaid and Swimming. In prone lengthening, the individual maintains a neutral TPC with light support upon their forearms as they activate the deep myofascial system and coordinate this with three-dimensional breathing.

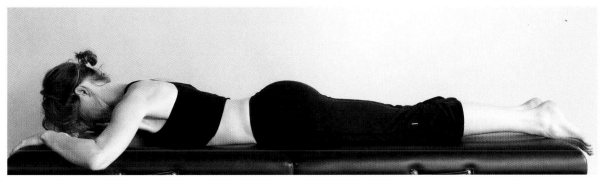

Figure 4.2: The prone lengthening position for developing core and scapular control.

Around the seventh to ninth month of life, continuing development of core stabilization and postural support enables a child to begin crawling (Figure 4.3). In addition to developing the core, crawling helps develop contralateral shoulder and hip stability, which is a prerequisite of upright support. The quadruped and crawling patterns help the transition into upright weight-bearing positions such as the squat (Figure 4.4).

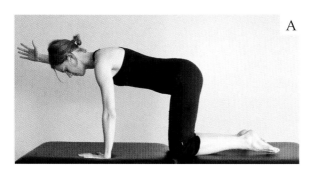
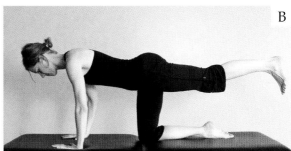

Figure 4.3: Crawling (left) and squat (right) patterns.

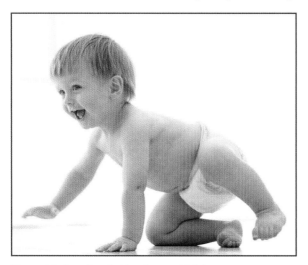
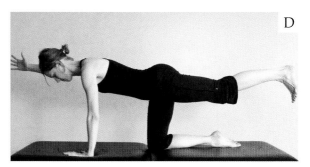
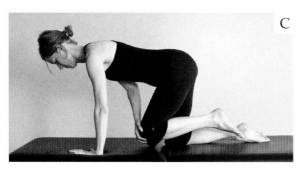

Figure 4.4: The Bird Dog exercise is an excellent pattern for developing core stability, with contralateral support and limb movement similar to the crawling pattern in Figure 4.3. While this is a common pattern in many rehabilitation programs, it is deceptively challenging to maintain a neutral TPC alignment while moving the limbs. To gain the most benefit from this pattern, be sure to progress the individual appropriately, ensuring that there is no movement of the spine or loss of shoulder control during the single limb lift (a-b) prior to performing the contralateral pattern (c-d).

At each moment of time within the first 12 to 15 months of life, the nervous system coordinates the myofascial, osseoligamentous, and respiratory systems in the process of achieving controlled upright posture and movement. With proper neuromotor development, a child will develop the stabilization strategies required to support upright posture and movement throughout life.

During this time, the nervous system develops the coordination of the myofascial system to support posture and movement through stereotypical patterns, such as supine, prone, rolling, crawling, and squatting. However, the development of optimal stabilization and movement can be disrupted if adequate time is not spent in developmental positions (supine, prone, etc.), or if artificial support aids are used to keep the child in a weight-bearing position before their osseous, myofascial, and ligamentous systems have developed the appropriate ability to support an upright posture (Figure 4.5).

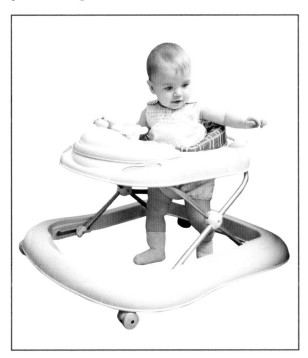

Figure 4.5: Disruption of the development of optimal stabilization and movement at an early age.

Dysfunction During Development

Professor Vaclav Vojta, a pediatric neurologist, was one of the early pioneers in developmental kinesiology, or the study of the neuromotor system during development. Professor Vojta worked with children with cerebral palsy and noted that healthy children responded to certain stimuli and possessed predictable, innate motor or muscle responses early in their development. He also recognized that these responses or reflexes were severely limited in children born with cerebral palsy.

Professor Vojta noted that activation of certain reflexive points and patterns of movement brought about improved motor response in his patients with cerebral palsy. From these findings, he developed the Vojta Principles, which formed the basis of Reflex Locomotion. Reflex Locomotion has influenced many pediatric and adult rehabilitation methods, including the Developmental Neuromuscular Stabilization model developed by Pavel Kolář.

Professor Vojta also noted that even among "healthy," or what were considered "normal," developing children, approximately one in three did not develop optimal neuromotor patterns (Cohen 2010). These children who develop inefficient stabilization and postural patterns have been characterized with central coordination disturbances, one of the primary causes of common postural alterations, including flat or over-pronated feet, valgus-knee (knock-knee) position, and winged scapula (Kolář et al. 2013).

Individuals with central coordination disturbances are likely to be less coordinated, or "clumsy," because they have not developed efficient or coordinated stabilization and movement strategies. These children are less likely to excel at athletics and often lag behind their classmates in basic running, jumping, throwing, or kicking ability. While this does not suggest that these children will necessarily develop more problems early on, it is likely that many of them will seek out movement specialists throughout their life, because they are prone to experience the deleterious effects related to their non-optimal postural and movement patterns.

Although these non-optimal patterns may be part of their lifelong nervous system programming, we can help these individuals improve their core stabilization strategy and movement patterns (Figure 4.6). The BAS, for example, is often extremely effective in developing and maintaining the fundamental core stabilization required to move towards improved function.

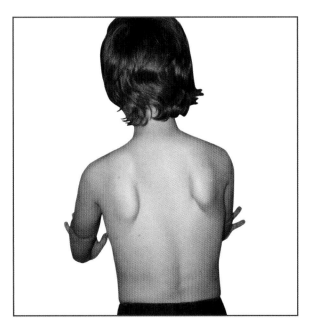
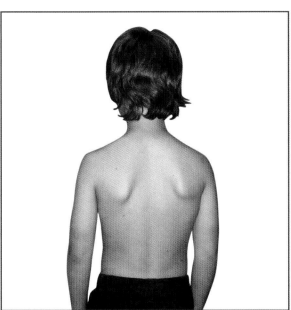

Figure 4.6: Winged scapula and excessive lumbar erector tone in a 10-year-old patient presenting with shoulder pain. These types of postural dysfunction that present at an early age are generally related to a non-optimal neural coordination of muscle activity. Adherence to the Pilates principles can help individuals with non-optimal stability strategies improve their postural and movement patterns.

Trauma

The second major reason for the development of core dysfunction is trauma. While acute trauma that occurs from a fall, motor vehicle accident, or contact injury can definitely affect core function, this section will focus primarily on repetitive trauma and surgery.

Repetitive Trauma

Repetitive traumas refer to the repetitive things we do every single day, as well as the way that

we perform these activities. These repetitive activities often lead to micro-traumas of the soft tissues of the body when they are performed with poor stabilization and/or beyond tissue tolerance. The micro-traumas may not necessarily create problems right away, but over time the cumulative effect will take its toll.

One of the most common culprits and best examples of micro-trauma in our modern society is sitting. Consider the length of time most of the population sit during the day. They sit to go to work, sit at work, and sit on the way home from work. Then at home, they sit while eating dinner or watching television before they go to bed. The bulk of their day is spent in the seated position.

Why does sitting have such a detrimental effect on our core function? While a significant part of the problem is related to the amount of time spent in a seated posture, many of the effects associated with sitting actually have to do with *how* these individuals are sitting.

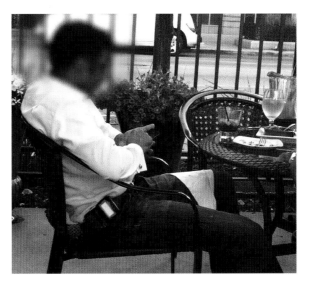

It is often said that increased sitting leads to common postural dysfunctions, such as an anterior pelvic tilt, and muscle imbalances that favor shortening of the hip flexors and lumbar erectors and over-lengthening of the glutes, hamstrings, and abdominals. However, is that really what happens? Note the common seated posture of individuals working on their laptop, playing video games, and sitting at a bar, for example (Figure 4.7). Each of these individuals is sitting in a posterior pelvic tilt with lumbar spine flexion. This is the posture assumed by most of our society when sitting during the majority of their day.

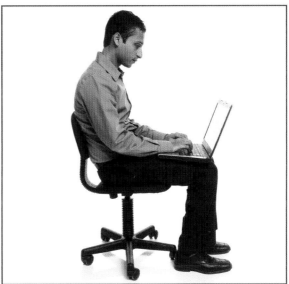

The underlying problem with the prolonged flexed sitting posture is that over time the soft tissue structures, including ligaments, joint capsules, and fascia, will slowly deform and elongate—a process referred to as *creep*. Prolonged flexion of the lumbar spine also causes the nucleus pulposus—the fluid-containing center of the disc—to migrate posteriorly. The posterior migration of the nucleus pulposus, combined with elongation of the supportive tissues, places the spinal discs in a disadvantaged position. This is a common cause of disc injury that eventually contributes to bulging and/or herniation.

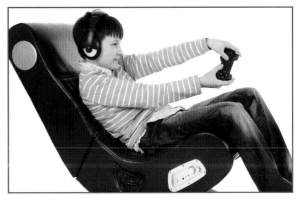

Figure 4.7: Whether looking at a phone, working on a laptop, or playing video games, the majority of us sit in posterior pelvic tilt with lumbar spine flexion. The biggest problem with this is that we spend too much time in this posture and tend not to move out of these flexed positions when standing up.

Moreover, with overstretching of these soft tissue structures there is less ability to stiffen the joint when required, placing the individual at a greater risk of joint instability and therefore of joint or soft tissue injury when postural loading is prolonged or as the tissues become more active. This is why an important part of our corrective strategy has to include teaching our clients how to sit more ideally, otherwise they may return to old patterns of sitting and can literally undo all the work they have done in their Pilates sessions.

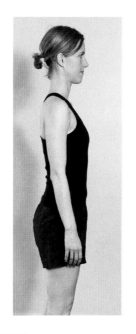
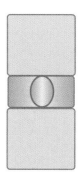

Figure 4.8: Spinal disc is well supported between the vertebrae with optimal postural alignment and balance of the myofascial systems.

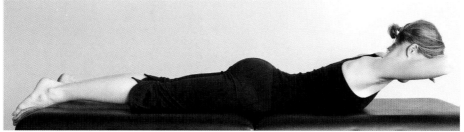
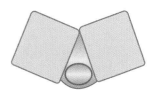

Figure 4.9: Nucleus pulposus moves anteriorly during Swan.

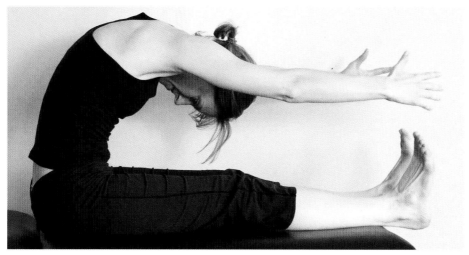
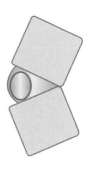

Figure 4.10: Nucleus pulposus shifts towards the back of the spine during spinal flexion.

With optimal postural alignment and balance of the myofascial systems, the spinal disc is well supported between the vertebrae (Figure 4.8). During Swan the spine moves into extension, and the nucleus pulposus moves anteriorly (Figure 4.9). However, during spinal flexion, as in the Roll-Up, the nucleus pulposus shifts towards the back of the spine (Figure 4.10). When individuals spend too much time in spinal flexion, and/or overdo spinal flexion exercises like Roll-Up, Teaser, and Hundreds, there is a potential for overstretching the posterior soft tissue structure and for disc injuries. This is especially common in individuals who spend much of their day sitting and/or standing in posterior pelvic tilt and lumbar spine flexion.

With optimal TPC control, the spine can remain stabilized even during flexion-based exercises, such as Up Stretch on the Reformer (Figure 4.11). When the hamstrings and posterior hip complex limit the range of anterior pelvic tilt, and/or the individual moves beyond their ability to stabilize their spine, the individual will compensate by flexing their spine. Note the loss of integrity in the spine (indicated by the arrow) during a forward fold (Figure 4.12). If continued, this habit will overstretch the posterior structures of the spine and increase the potential for low back and disc issues.

There is another phenomenon that occurs in the soft tissues with prolonged or repetitive soft tissue loading. *Hysteresis* refers to ligament, joint capsule, and fascial lengthening that occurs with repetitive loading. It is a normal phenomenon during activities such as bending forward, chopping wood, or performing a Pilates Roll-Up.

The problem arises when individuals who are fixed in a posterior pelvic tilt and lumbar flexion perform repetitive flexion-based activities. These individuals tend to perpetuate

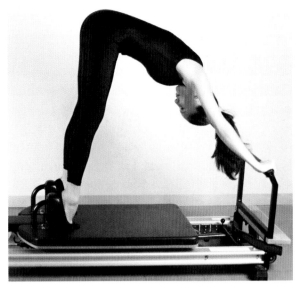

Figure 4.11: Up Stretch on the Reformer.

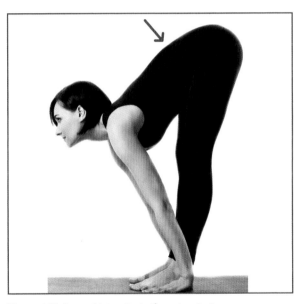

Figure 4.12: Loss of integrity in the spine during a forward fold.

their muscle imbalances if they perform too many flexion-based exercises without first developing a more ideal core stabilization strategy. This is also why so many core exercise programs fail to help people develop optimal core function; many exercise programs are not training these individuals in a manner that helps them find and control neutral alignment. This is where Pilates training and incorporating the six principles can be so valuable in helping to correct chronic muscle imbalances and move towards establishing a more efficient core stabilization strategy that supports optimal posture and movement.

A Few Words About Spinal Flexion

It is important to note that spinal flexion is a requirement of life and therefore should not be avoided. However, we need to ensure that our core is aligned and that we have developed control before adding in flexion-based movements, so that we can handle the stress of repetitive flexion. This is a major reason why the respiratory retraining and core stabilization strategy presented earlier focused so much on improving control of the neutral TPC alignment and on how to activate the deep myofascial system. Developing balance between the deep and superficial myofascial systems and teaching control of neutral alignment of the TPC enable our core system to meet the demands of life.

Another reason why spinal flexion exercises are contraindicated before an individual has developed an optimal core stabilization strategy is the stresses placed on the spine during these types of exercise. Spinal flexion exercises, such as the Pilates Roll-Up, train the core in a relatively flexed spine position. Historically, some schools of Pilates have taught an imprinted spine during supine abdominal exercises, such as the Ab Series (Single-Leg Stretch, Double-Leg Stretch,

Criss-Cross, Lower Lift), the Hundred, and others. Flattening, or imprinting, reduces the curvature in your spine, which is essentially causing spinal flexion. While not a problem for individuals with a well-stabilized core, this can pose a problem for those having posterior pelvic tilt and lumbar spine flexion, and experiencing the effects of creep and hysteresis. This is why we initially stress control of neutral thoracopelvic alignment and ensure that we can control this alignment (by keeping the head down on the mat) before adding spinal flexion, such as chest lifting or imprinting. Learn also to maintain a neutral lumbar spine during spinal flexion in other planes of gravity, not just in supine. In a seated position, Spine Stretch Forward, Saw, Short Box, and Stomach Massage are excellent exercises to develop the ability to control.

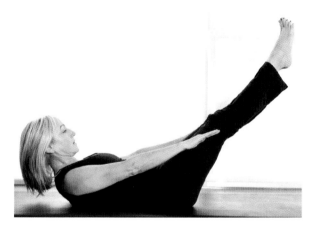

Figure 4.13: Hundreds pattern.

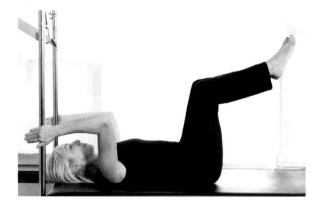

Figure 4.14: Table Top position.

For individuals lacking control of neutral TPC alignment, the Hundreds pattern can create low back and pelvic problems (Figure 4.13). It is important to establish neutral control of the TPC with patterns such as the Table Top position before adding in flexion-based exercise (Figure 4.14).

Don't Just Sit There!
After looking through the histories of nearly 100,000 individuals, a revealing prospective study of the detrimental effects of sitting concluded that people who sat more than six hours a day had a 40 percent increased risk of premature death, compared with those who sat for less than three hours (Patel et al. 2010). Furthermore, it was suggested that even intense exercise is not enough to undo these risk factors if the individual still spends the bulk of their day sitting. However, taking short breaks—such as getting out of the chair and moving around every hour, adjusting the posture, and doing some deep diaphragmatic breathing—has anecdotally helped make a positive change in many of our clients who have to sit for work. If you are a Pilates instructor, encourage your clients to move a lot during their day!

Surgery

Another common, and often understated, cause of trauma to the body is surgery. Every surgical procedure is a traumatic event for the body, and no surgery should be considered "routine" or free of side effects. Any time the myofascial system is cut through, even with small external incisions, internal scar tissue will form as part of the healing cascade.

Although laparoscopic surgery has less visible scarring and less cutting of superficial muscle, there is still significant cutting of supportive fascia beneath the surface, which often leads to significant scar tissue. While there are only three small sites of entry into the abdomen during laparoscopic surgery, in order to better see during the procedure the abdominal cavity is filled with gas, thereby further disrupting the deep intramuscular and intravisceral fascial systems (the latter surrounds and supports the organs). This can also create post-surgical fascial adhesions not only around the actual entry site, but in the surrounding abdominal and visceral fascia as well.

As noted, all surgery creates scar tissue and the more significant the surgery, generally the greater the scar tissue. Dr. Jean Claude Guimberteau, a hand and wrist surgeon, has done incredible work to demonstrate the fluidity of healthy fascia. His research has demonstrated that scar tissue forms at the surgical site less than three months after surgery and affects the natural fluidity and gliding function of the fascia, even within this short time frame (Guimberteau 2012). Think about the individuals who have had surgery 10, 20, or even 30 years ago, or multiple surgeries over a number of years, and how much scar tissue and compensations can occur during that time.

Case in Point

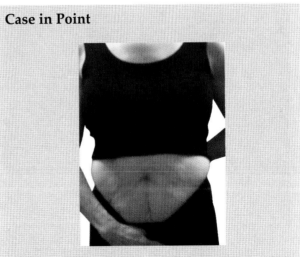

Figure 4.15: Complications caused by the formation of scar tissue following a cesarean.

The woman in Figure 4.15 is a patient of Evan's who had her only child via cesarean section; although she had significant low back pain, she reported no abdominal or gastrointestinal (GI) issues for five years post-delivery. Then she began experiencing intestinal pain and was rushed into emergency for surgery—hence this vertical scar. The surgeon discovered that scar tissue which formed after her initial surgery had strangulated her intestines and, as a result, she had to have a section of her GI tract removed. Additionally, the surgeon noted there was scar tissue formation that had attached from her abdominal wall straight through to her sacrum.

We added the example of the woman with post-cesarean formation of scar tissue to impress upon you that a large portion of our client and patient population has had abdominal surgery, whether it is cesarean section, hysterectomy, cholecystectomy (gall bladder removal), ovarian cyst removal, or gastrointestinal resection. We have seen a significant portion of our population who have developed significant scar tissue and have compromised function, especially of their deep myofascial system. The more time that has passed, the more complicated the corrective surgery, and the greater the number of surgeries the individual has had, the more likely the development of increased compensations to their core stabilization strategy. These compensations lead directly to postural and movement dysfunction (Lee and Lee 2013, Wetzler 2014, Osar 2014).

Special Note to Pilates Instructors
How can we best help individuals who have had surgery of the trunk, abdominal wall, pelvis, and/or low back? First, inquire about their surgical history to determine whether it seems relevant to their current postural and/or movement issues. Many of these individuals will need to be evaluated by a specialized manual therapist who can assess for deeper scar tissue as well as visceral mobility (movement of the organs within their fascial environment). We have found that individuals with prior surgery often require specific scar tissue mobilization from a qualified therapist in addition to release of the over-activity within the superficial myofascial system as a result of it compensating for inhibition of the deep system. Additionally, by aligning the TPC, activating the deep myofascial system, and incorporating three-dimensional breathing, you can help restore mobility to the deep and superficial fascial systems, including the fascia surrounding their abdominal and pelvic organs. And by integrating this function into Pilates exercises, you will help many people return to more normalized posture and movement.

For more information on visceral mobilization and the effects of scar tissue upon the visceral system visit: http://www.barralinstitute.com/.

Habituation

The third category that leads to core dysfunction and becomes a real challenge to developing and/or maintaining optimal core function is habituation. You can think of habituation as the repetitive ways we have done things through the course of our life that have created, and continue to influence, our ability to stabilize and move. Let's look at a few of these habits that can dramatically affect core stabilization and significantly alter our movement patterns.

One of the most common habits we have learned through the course of our life is our postural strategy. We will discuss several variations of common postural habits that strongly influence core stability (Figure 4.16).

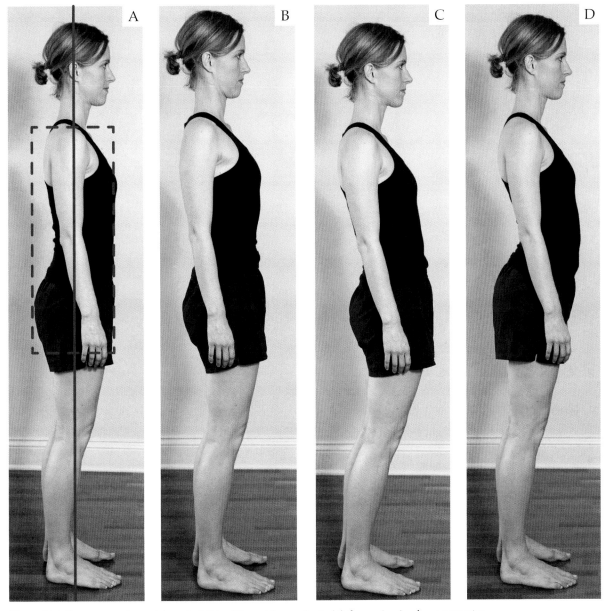

Figure 4.16: Common postures: (a) neutral; (b) military; (c) sway back; (d) thoracolumbar hyperextension.

Neutral Posture

In neutral posture, the thorax is aligned over the pelvis, there is maintenance of the spinal curvature, and, when viewed from the side, an imaginary plumb line extends through the ear, cervical and lumbar spines, down through the knee joint, to a point just anterior to the ankle joint. This posture promotes optimal three-dimensional breathing and activation of the deep myofascial system, as well as encouraging length in the superficial myofascial chains. Note that this model's posture is, in fact, slightly pitched forward, not a true neutral alignment. This is due to factors outside the scope of this book and may be corrected with awareness and/or structural bodywork.

Military Posture

Individuals presenting with a military posture tend to hold their body very rigid. There is over-activation of the neck flexors, abdominals, and glutes, and hence there tends to be a loss of spinal curvature in all three regions of the spine—cervical, thoracic, and lumbar. These individuals commonly hold their thorax behind their pelvis, and the pelvis exhibits a posterior pelvic tilt. This rigid and braced type of strategy makes it nearly impossible to develop optimal three-dimensional breathing and consequently there is heavy reliance on a bracing strategy for core stability.

Sway Back Posture

In sway back posture, the individual tends to hang off the soft tissue structures of their anterior hip. They generally have shortening of the rectus abdominis, with shallowness of the anterior thorax. Shortening of the rectus abdominis limits the ability to elevate the anterior thorax during inspiration, so such individuals tend to be primarily belly breathers. They will also tend to hold their thorax behind their pelvis, which, combined with overstretching of the lower abdominals, compromises their ability to stabilize their core.

Thoracolumbar Hyperextension Posture

Thoracolumbar hyperextension is an increasingly common postural alignment, especially among exercise enthusiasts, including yoga and Pilates practitioners. This posture is most often caused by cueing that encourages the individual to lift their ribcage up and pull their shoulder blades into retraction (down and back). Thoracolumbar hyperextension is characterized by over-activity in the thoracolumbar erectors and

the subsequent increase in extension at the thoracolumbar (TL) junction. Excessive TL extension inhibits posterolateral breathing, and these individuals are unable therefore to activate the deep myofascial system, especially where the TVA, diaphragm, psoas, and quadratus lumborum myofascially blend into the TL junction. These individuals will also tend to be belly breathers, as the increased myofascial erector tone inhibits posterior breathing. As a consequence, these individuals will be unable to appropriately generate the IAP required to support loading, so they will have to over-rely on a bracing strategy for support. The excessive extension also overstretches the anterior abdominal wall, creating an increased potential for abdominal or sports hernias and increased pressure into the pelvic floor. Additionally, these individuals often report chronic back stiffness or tightness because of their non-optimal strategy. For many of these individuals, simply developing a more efficient core stabilization strategy, and cueing them out of these non-optimal postural habits, will eliminate much of their chronic tightness.

One of my (Evan's) patients reported with complaints of shoulder pain and chronic headaches (Figure 4.17). She demonstrated a common postural pattern of a long lordosis from her low back to her upper thorax. This posture tends to make the thorax (ribcage and thoracic spine) very stiff, especially through the posterior aspect, making it nearly impossible for the individual to perform three-dimensional breathing. This limitation ultimately affects their ability to develop intra-abdominal pressure and stabilize the core. Interestingly, this patient reported that from the time she was a little girl, her mother instructed her to lift her chest and pull her shoulder blades down and back, illustrating how many of our habits today have been set up by things we learned many years ago.

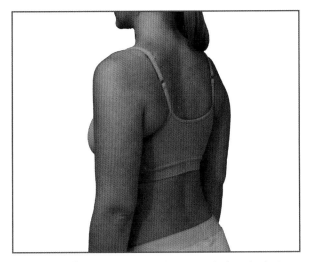

Figure 4.17: The common postural pattern of a long lordosis from the low back to the upper thorax.

Many older individuals tend to have increased thoracic kyphosis and likewise hold their thorax behind their pelvis. As with several of the aforementioned postures, they also commonly present with a posterior pelvic tilt from over-activation of their posterior hip complex—in Figure 4.18 note the decreased mass in this man's gluteal region from years of chronic hip gripping.

These types of alteration can occur in anyone who adopts and maintains a certain posture for an extended period of time—as most of us tend to do. This again illustrates why it is so important to improve an individual's postural strategy through improved core stabilization and to educate them on ways of adopting more ideal habits.

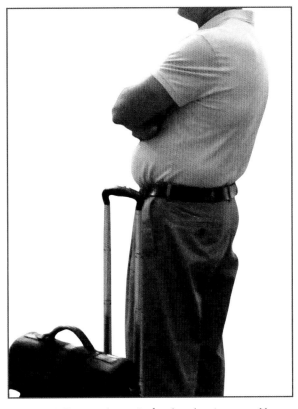

Figure 4.18: Decreased mass in the gluteal region caused by years of chronic hip gripping.

Over-activation of the Abdominal Wall

Another common and often associated pattern contributing to non-optimal postural and movement strategies is over-activation of the abdominal wall. Despite what well-meaning parents and teachers instructed, we should not pull our stomachs in or hold the abdominal wall "tight" or contracted for most of the day. Not only is this a dysfunctional core stabilization strategy, but also over-activation of the abdominal wall will inhibit three-dimensional breathing and the development of an efficient core stabilization strategy. Because its attachments span from the anterior ribcage to the pelvis, contracting the abdominal wall will typically flatten the lumbar curvature and pull the pelvis into a posterior pelvic tilt (Figure 4.19). This leads to a reduction or flexion of the lumbar spine.

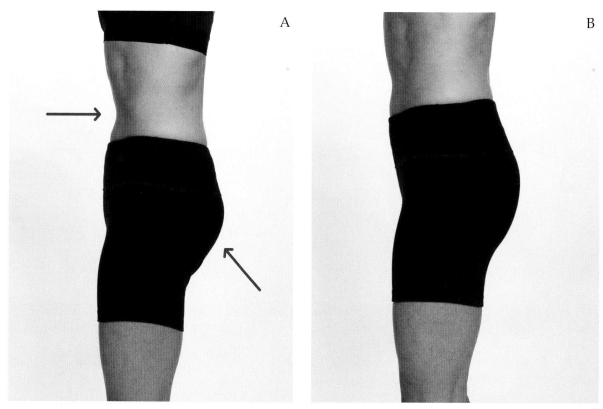

Figure 4.19: (a) Note the individual holding her stomach tight by abdominal hollowing. She also grips her posterior hip region, which, combined with increased abdominal activation, pulls her into lumbar spine flexion and a posterior pelvic tilt. (b) With a verbal cue to think long and relax her abdominal wall and posterior hip complex, she achieves more neutral alignment of her spine and pelvis.

This does not mean the abdominal wall should not be toned: it just means we should not live our lives with a perpetually contracted abdomen. Just as you would not walk around with your arms flexed all day, you should not walk around with your abdominals contracted all the time, either. Living each day with our abdominals pulled in may look nice aesthetically, but it is a dysfunctional strategy for postural control.

The need or the habit of overly activating the superficial abdominal wall (obliques and rectus abdominis) is a common stabilization strategy for several reasons, including:

• Inhibition of the deep abdominal wall secondary to surgery, as discussed above.
• Abdominal distension (lower abdominal bulge), which occurs secondary to an inflamed gastrointestinal tract (chronic inflammatory bowel disease or inflammation that occurs as a result of over-consumption of dairy, wheat, sugar, and other common food allergens).
• Being self-conscious of excessive abdominal fat and either knowingly or unknowingly drawing in or hollowing the abdominal wall to diminish the appearance of the midsection.

Regardless of the cause, over-activation of the abdominal wall leads to core dysfunction. Teaching optimal breathing and core activation as we discussed in Chapter 3 will enable you or your client to develop more integrated abdominal function and thus a more functional—and slimmer—midsection.

When we have ideal or neutral posture, our joints are aligned and we breathe optimally, and we do not have the need or desire to excessively brace or hang off our soft tissue structures. We are balanced and can easily maintain upright alignment without the need for compensatory positions. It is important that individuals with postural alterations are taught a more optimal core stabilization strategy as well as more ideal postural habits, or they will likely return to their habitual patterns, thereby negating the improvements we are attempting to create through training.

Exercise Habituation

Many common exercises can perpetuate core dysfunction as well. Though effective at strengthening the back, when performed without regard to the development of TPC stability and optimal respiratory patterns the hyperextension and reverse hyperextension patterns can lead to increasing levels of core dysfunction (Figure 4.20). Without the ability to stabilize the anterior abdominal wall and lengthen the spine either during trunk extension (hyperextension) or when the legs are lifted (reverse hyperextension), an individual will tend to hyperextend where the spine is most mobile. In many, it is common for this extension to occur at the thoracolumbar junction (region where the thoracic spine meets the lumbar spine), perpetuating the thoracolumbar hyperextension posture and inhibiting optimal core function.

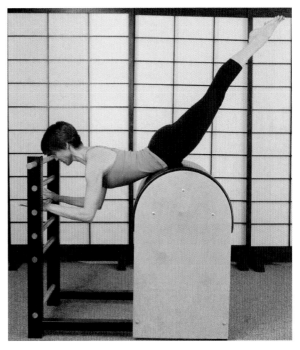

Figure 4.20: Swan on the Barrel. Without balance between the myofascial systems, these extension-dominant patterns will over-activate the thoracolumbar erectors and prevent posterior diaphragmatic breathing. Loss of posterolateral breathing inhibits development of intra-abdominal pressure, resulting in over-compression of the posterior ribcage and lumbar spine.

Stretching without control can also contribute to a loss of TPC stabilization. Note the loss of TPC connection and resultant thoracolumbar hyperextension in the woman stretching her hip flexors (Figure 4.21(a)). This strategy for stretching will cause overstretching of the psoas and anterior abdominal wall, thereby perpetuating core dysfunction. Controlling her TPC while maintaining connection between her thorax and pelvis, Marylee is able to stretch her hip flexors without compromising stability (Figure 4.21(b)). Maintaining integrity of the TPC while stretching is the safest way to simultaneously achieve flexibility and stability.

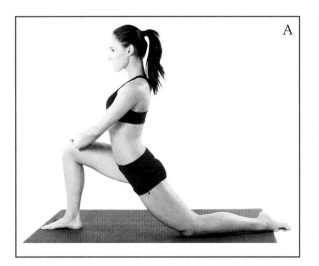
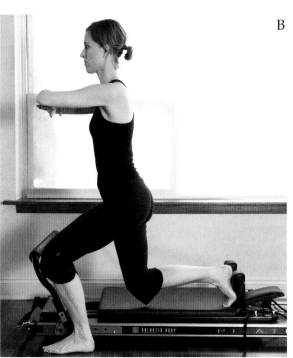

Figure 4.21: Stretching the hip flexors: (a) loss of TPC connection and resultant thoracolumbar hyperextension; (b) control of the TPC while maintaining connection between the thorax and the pelvis.

Conclusion

In this chapter we have covered three common reasons why we develop core dysfunction. Each of these affects our system in a different way depending on our unique development as a child, medical history, exercise and occupation choices, and messages that we give our body throughout our life. They are as follows:

1. Neurodevelopmental: In individuals where there are non-optimal neuromotor programs during childhood development, stabilization and movement patterns become delayed and/or inhibited, resulting in compensated stabilization and postural strategies that are reflected in adult posture and movement.

2. Trauma: Trauma has a deep and profound effect on our system, whether it occurs from surgery or whether it is other acute or repetitive trauma. Most traumas, especially surgery, create muscle inhibition and compensatory patterns; the more significant and long-lasting the muscle inhibition, the more challenging it is to change those behaviors.

Habits: For many of us, our habits dictate how we stabilize, hold our posture, and move. These habits have been formed by the exercises we perform, the cues we follow during exercise, the internal messages we tell ourselves about our body, and what we consider to be normal function and how we perform it. These habits form the basis of how we stand, sit, sleep, work, and play. Each category contributes to non-optimal respiratory patterns, myofascial imbalances, and inefficient stabilization strategies that cause postural, and eventually movement, dysfunction. It is these resultant dysfunctional patterns that lead to the chronic tightness, pain syndromes, and degenerative joint conditions experienced by so many people. In the next chapter we look at how the nervous system compensates for these inefficient strategies.

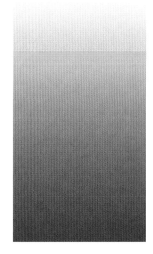

Responses to Non-optimal Core Stabilization Strategies

5

Having covered the three primary causes of core dysfunction in Chapter 4, we will now look at the signs and systemic effects of these non-efficient strategies. Unfortunately, core dysfunction is not easily detected by what an individual cannot do, because many of us perform at a relatively high level even with inefficient core stabilization strategies. This chapter will identify and explore some of the common signs and systemic effects of poor core stabilization, as well as the compensatory patterns we adopt as a result of the dysfunction.

In this chapter you will discover:

- How non-optimal strategies affect the nervous system
- The development of imbalances and the compensations of the deep and superficial myofascial systems
- The three gripping strategies an individual might adopt to compensate for the loss of control

Effect on the Autonomic Nervous System

In review, the autonomic nervous system is the part of the nervous system that regulates body functions, such as heart rate, digestion, respiratory rate, and sexual function. It consists of two main divisions: the sympathetic and the parasympathetic nervous systems. When our body is optimally functioning—meaning that we feel good, we are eating and resting well, our mood is positive, and we have efficient stabilization and movement strategies—the sympathetic (fight-or-flight) and parasympathetic (rest-and-digest) parts of the nervous system are in balance.

However, when an imbalance is created between these two systems—as can occur with inadequate sleep and recuperation, exercising too much relative to the amount of rest, anxiety, stress, and/or trauma—there tends to be an increase in the sympathetic nervous system activity. The most significant result of sympathetic nervous system predominance, and what ultimately leads to a poor core stabilization strategy, is the impact on our respiratory system.

When an individual has shifted primarily to a sympathetic-dominant breathing strategy there are several indications and characteristic stereotypes that will be noted:

• Their breathing cycles begin to shorten, because they have shifted to using an upper-chest and neck breathing strategy, rather than using the diaphragm and primary muscles of respiration. Along with an elevated ribcage position that results from chronic use of this upper airway breathing strategy, the shortened breathing cycle also limits their ability to fully expire air. We have clinically observed that these individuals will "sigh" in an attempt to lower their ribcage and expel air.

• Because of the increasing stiffness of the thorax and the subsequent decreasing ability to fully expire air from their lungs, the individual's breaths become increasingly shallow. As a consequence of the resultant poor oxygenation and circulation, they will increase the rate or frequency of their respiratory cycles to meet the body's demand for oxygen and waste removal. Simply increasing the number of breaths per minute from 8–12 to 13–20 means that the amount of work that needs to be done by the accessory muscles of respiration is increased by virtually 60 percent over the course of one day. Consider the increase in the amount of work that the myofascial system has to do over the course of many years of using this strategy.

• To meet the demands, the individual will often overuse the scalenes, sterno-cleidomastoid, and pectoralis minor to expand the thoracic dimensions by elevating the upper ribs, sternum, and clavicles. This leads to chronic stiffness and shortness in these muscles and is perhaps the most common cause of the forward-head and forward-shoulder positions. In addition to their effect on respiration, these chronically shortened muscles tend to contribute to both neck and shoulder issues.

• The cumulative effects of this dysfunctional respiratory strategy are increased anxiety, irritability, and chronic fatigue, which then perpetuate the cycle.

As this respiratory dysfunction develops into a self-perpetuating cycle (Figure 5.1), it begins to alter how the individual stabilizes their core: without being able to take optimal three-dimensional breaths, they are unable to develop adequate levels of intra-abdominal pressure to stabilize and decompress their trunk. Recall that intra-abdominal pressure has the dual purpose of providing stability and decreasing the combination of gravity, bodyweight, external loads, and ground reaction forces that compress the trunk, spine, and pelvis.

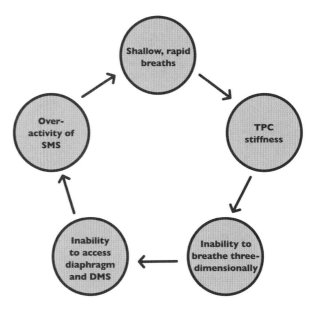

Figure 5.1: Perpetuating cycle of breathing and core dysfunction.

Effect on Posture and the Deep Myofascial System

While a faulty breathing strategy leads to the obvious systemic effects of poor oxygenation and circulation, a more relevant issue related to function is that it sets the individual up for having non-optimal core stabilization strategies. This occurs because of the postural alterations and their impact on myofascial activity.

As we discussed in Chapter 4, a common sign of respiratory dysfunction is a significant ribcage flare as the thorax becomes fixated or "stuck" in the inspiratory position (Figure 5.2). This position is characterized by an increase in the sternal–costal angle and prominence of the lower anterior ribcage.

This alignment also leads to overstretching of the anterior abdominal wall and can often result in the development of a condition called *diastasis recti* (splitting of the two halves of the rectus abdominis). Although this is common during pregnancy as a result of the growth of the child and stretching of the abdominal wall, it is often found in people with poor respiratory patterns, where the diaphragm and ribcage are held in an inspiratory position, which overstretches and functionally inhibits the abdominal wall. As a result of a non-optimal breathing strategy combined with overstretching of the abdominal wall, more pressure is pushed down into the abdominal and pelvic cavities, further inhibiting the abdominal wall. The resultant pull of the oblique abdominals creates a separation of the rectus abdominis.

Though it can be visible on those who have a very lean abdominal wall, diastasis recti is usually detected by palpating between the two halves of the rectus abdominis: as the individual performs a crunching motion,

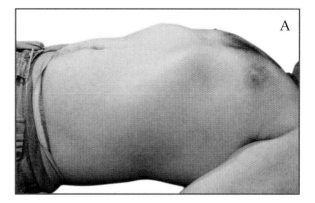

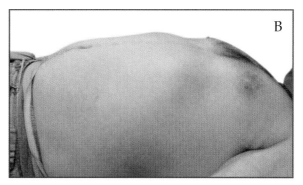

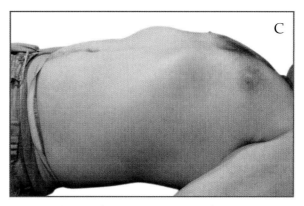

Figure 5.2: (a) Note the wide angle between the lower anterior ribs and prominence with non-optimal alignment and rigidity of the TPC; (b) during inspiration this client demonstrates a good abdominal breathing strategy; (c) because of thoracic rigidity, however, he cannot bring his anterior ribs inferiorly during expiration and therefore maintains an inspiratory position of the ribcage, which will limit his ability to generate optimal levels of IAP and lead to overuse of his superficial myofascial system for support. Additionally, this non-optimal breathing strategy will perpetuate thoracic rigidity and is a common cause of low back tightness as well as of shoulder and hip dysfunction.

your fingers will drop through the split in the abdominal wall and into their abdomen. It is important that these individuals are taught an optimal activation strategy that encourages the deep muscles (primarily the transversus abdominis and investing abdominal fascia) to hold the rectus abdominis closed during their Pilates exercises. Often it is not advisable to perform flexion-based exercises (Roll-Ups, Teasers, Hundreds, etc.) until they can maintain a connected or "closed" rectus abdominis position.

Even individuals who appear fit but have performed too many flexion-based abdominal exercises with a poor breathing and stabilization strategy are at risk of developing diastasis recti. Note the separation of the rectus abdominis in the bodybuilder in Figure 5.3. You can often see the diastasis recti as the individual performs trunk flexion; you will notice the abdominal organs pushing up through the split of the rectus abdominis. It is important that these clients are instructed how to control their diastasis recti and develop an improved core stabilization strategy.

Pelvic floor dysfunction can be another common sign of poor respiratory and core stabilization strategy. Stress incontinence, an involuntary loss of urine while exercising, coughing, sneezing, or laughing affects about one in three females, or almost 25 million women in America, with higher rates for women who have had children, the elderly, and men who have had prostate surgery. Moreover, this problem is not limited to these groups. A study done on elite college athletes found that almost one third of female athletes experienced urinary incontinence. The average age of the women in these studies was 20 and none had gone through childbirth. Twenty-eight percent reported urine loss while participating in their sport; two thirds of the women who were incontinent reported

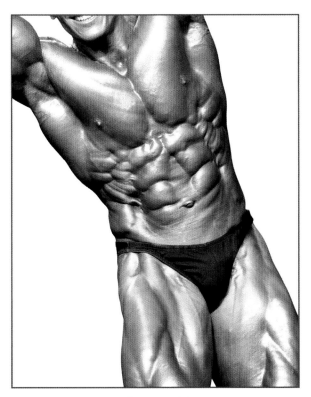

Figure 5.3: Separation of the rectus abdominis in a bodybuilder.

that it was a regular occurrence, and 40 percent first noticed these symptoms in junior high or high school (Nygarrd et al. 1994).

In another study, researchers looked at different sitting postures and the effects these had on pelvic floor activity in continent and incontinent women (Sapsford et al. 2008). They evaluated slumped-supported, upright-unsupported, and very tall, unsupported postures and their effects on the activation of the pelvic floor. Neutral pelvic positioning in the upright, unsupported position increased resting pelvic floor muscle activity in both continent and incontinent women. Interestingly, it was also noted that continent women tended to have increased lordotic curvatures in unsupported upright sitting, compared with the incontinent women. This is another reason why we advocate beginning training in neutral pelvic and spinal postures before moving clients on to other positions:

in this way, activation of the deep myofascial system is improved, and the least amount of stress tends to be placed on the spine and pelvis in individuals who may currently have issues (Figure 5.4).

Another problem that stems from the wide-anterior or inspiratory-fixed position of the ribcage is gastroesophageal reflux disease (GERD). GERD occurs when the gastric, or stomach, acid leaks up into the esophagus, causing irritation of the esophageal lining. It is estimated that GERD affects nearly one in three individuals, and over $10 billion is spent annually in the United States treating this problem. One overlooked cause of GERD is a non-optimal breathing strategy.

The esophagus passes through the diaphragm, and contraction of the diaphragm helps regulate closure of the esophageal sphincter, preventing regurgitation of stomach acid into the esophagus. When the diaphragm is fixed or stuck because of an inspiratory position of the ribcage, as is the case in the majority of our patients and clients with dysfunctional breathing, it is less effective at aiding closure of the esophageal sphincter. Breathing exercises have been shown to improve gastroesophageal reflux disease (Eherer et al. 2012), again demonstrating how optimizing our breathing strategy can have a direct and significant impact on our entire system.

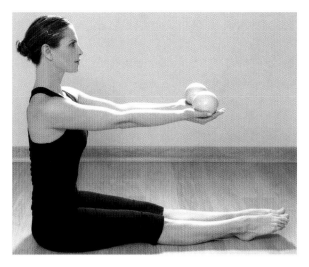

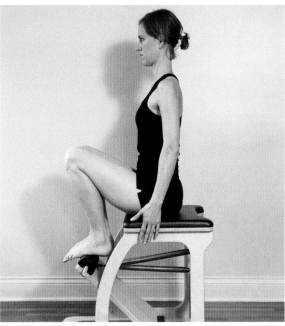

Figure 5.4: Developing control of neutral alignment of the TPC improves activation of the deep myofascial system, allowing better control of posture and movement. For those who lack the requisite hip flexion or control to maintain this position while sitting on the floor, the wunda chair provides an excellent alternative.

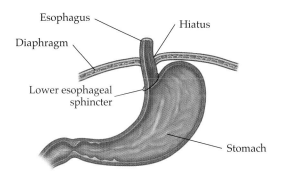

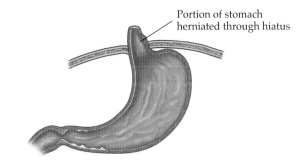

Figure 5.5: The esophagus passes through the diaphragm, and contraction of the diaphragm helps regulate closure of the esophageal sphincter, preventing regurgitation of stomach acid into the esophagus.

Compensatory Strategies for the Lack of Optimal Control

In Chapter 4 we looked at the three main causes of the development of dysfunctional core stabilization: neurodevelopment, trauma, and habits. In that chapter we discussed some of the common systemic effects as well as the signs indicating that an individual has developed a dysfunctional core strategy. We will now look at how the nervous system deals with the loss of an optimal core stabilization strategy and some of the common compensations adopted by an individual when they have developed non-optimal breathing and core stabilization strategies.

Recall that our body is subject to the same gravitational forces and biomechanical properties that all static structures, such as buildings, are exposed to. However, unlike a static building, we do not just bend or crumble to the ground when something is not working properly. To our advantage, the nervous system is very adept at compensating to accomplish our functional tasks of life. For example:

• When we are exposed to forces our body has not been trained to handle—like learning a new skill such as swinging a golf club—the nervous system is able to coordinate muscle activity that allows us to carry on participating, even if, for instance, the swing is inefficient.
• When lifting a weight that is heavier than what our core can actually stabilize, the nervous system can over-recruit certain muscles to help us accomplish the task.
• When our muscles have fatigued and we ought to stop exercising but we keep going regardless during an intense Pilates exercise class or during a long run, for example, our nervous system allows us to push through this phase by using compensatory strategies and/or muscle recruitment.

Ideally, when there is co-activation of the muscle synergists around a joint, we can control joint centration (alignment and control of the joint position) during functional activity without compensation. For example, the deep, lower fibers of the gluteus maximus, along with the psoas, are functional antagonists that help centrate the femoral head within the acetabulum (Figure 5.6). With optimal core stabilization and muscle activation, the femoral head will remain centrated within the acetabulum, while the pelvis and lumbar spine will remain aligned and controlled during hip extension.

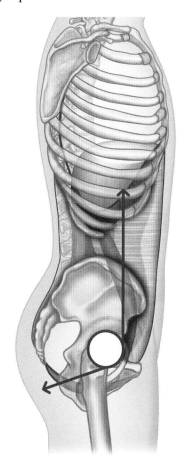

Figure 5.6: The deep, lower fibers of the gluteus maximus, along with the psoas, help centrate the femoral head within the acetabulum.

However, it is common for the gluteus maximus and psoas to become inhibited and lose their capacity to centrate the hip and contribute optimally in hip extension. In particular, the lower fibers of the gluteus maximus are part of the deep myofascial system and, along with the psoas, draw or pull the femoral head posteriorly into the acetabulum, thereby helping maintain an aligned and controlled hip joint and allowing optimal hip extension (Gibbons 2005).

When the lower, medial gluteal fibers or deep fibers of the psoas are inhibited and fail to optimally maintain centration of the femoral head within the acetabulum, the hamstrings, as synergists to hip extension, increase their activity (Figure 5.7). Since the hamstrings are part of the superficial myofascial system and lie further from the axis of joint rotation, they are unable to maintain joint centration. As the hamstrings contract, they drive the femoral head anteriorly in the acetabulum. It is also common for individuals who lack hip-extension force to compensate by excessively anteriorly tilting the pelvis and hyperextending the lumbar spine (Figure 5.8(c)).

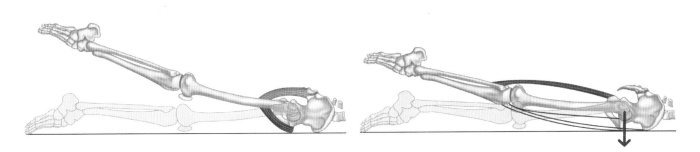

Figure 5.7: With optimal balance between the myofascial systems the hip remains centrated during hip extension (left). With loss of deep myofascial control the hamstrings can become dominant as hip extensors and drive the femoral head anteriorly during hip extension (right).

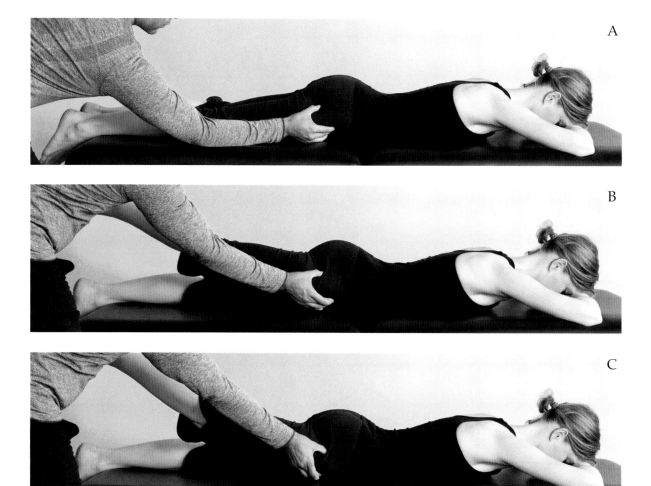

A

B

C

Figure 5.8. During Pilates exercises, such as Swimming or Double-Leg Kick, we want to extend our hips while controlling a neutral hip position and maintaining relative neutral alignment of the pelvis and lumbar spine. Note in images (a) and (b) how Marylee is able to maintain optimal joint centration when the myofascial systems are balanced. Palpation reveals that the femoral head remains centrated and there is no change in pelvic alignment. When there is muscle imbalance and increased activity of the hamstrings, the individual compensates by driving the femoral head forward within the acetabulum and/or excessively anteriorly rotating the pelvis. In this case, palpation shows the femoral head being excessively driven forward when there is loss of hip centration, as seen in image (c).

Additionally, because of their reduced ability to extend their hip, these individuals will generally compensate by excessively anteriorly rotating the pelvis and/or extending the low back, creating pseudo hip extension. Then, as they walk, run, or exercise, instead of being able to maintain a long spine and control their lower extremity, as they go into hip extension the pelvis rotates excessively into anterior rotation and/or the femoral head is driven forward in the acetabulum or the lumbar spine

excessively extends. Often a combination of all three of these compensatory patterns occurs, which is one of the more common scenarios that lead to hip, sacroiliac joint, and/or low back pain, and tightness in runners.

Understand and Apply
Having an understanding of functional anatomy not only helps us understand why we develop problems, but, more importantly, also allows us to develop a strategy for improving

our stabilization and movement patterns on the basis of nervous system function. By understanding and applying this knowledge we can develop strategies that enable us to stabilize and move with greater efficiency and less likelihood of dysfunction.

The above scenario where the hamstrings are substituting for an inhibited gluteus maximus is a classic example of synergist dominance. *Synergist dominance* occurs when there is inhibition of the prime movers, and the synergist muscles take over the primary role of the movement. In this case, inhibition of the gluteus maximus (prime mover) led to the hamstrings (synergists) assuming the primary role of hip extension.

Similarly, when there is inhibition of the deep myofascial system and joint integrity or control is compromised, the superficial myofascial system increases its activity to help provide an increased level of joint stability. In response to trauma or joint inflammation that creates inhibition of the deep myofascial system, the superficial myofascial system becomes synergistically dominant in joint stabilization. A synergistically dominant superficial myofascial system is a typical compensatory strategy for dealing with muscle inhibition and/or compromised joint centration.

In other words, a common response of the nervous system to deal with an inefficient stabilization strategy is to over-contract the myofascial system. To illustrate this strategy, think about your reaction to walking over a slippery surface. What is your nervous system's reaction to any unstable environment, such as walking over a slippery tile floor or on ice? Do you walk tall with long, confident strides? Or do you tend to walk slower, more methodically, with more flexion and even adduction in your limbs? Of course—the

latter is the most common response to our nervous system detecting and compensating for unstable conditions.

The nervous system reacts by tightening regions of the body to create increased levels of stability, which is generally the preferred response when there is muscle inhibition. This strategy is what enabled our ancestors to hunt, forage, travel, lift, build, and fight off their enemies, even in the presence of muscle inhibition. Without this compensatory ability, we would probably not be here to write this book and you would not be here to read it; we would have fallen prey to a hungry animal or victim during a battle.

However, there is one major caveat to this strategy: it is a good strategy except when we are unable to let go of it, or when it becomes our predominant go-to means of stabilization. We refer to this compensatory strategy of over-tightening or over-contracting the myofascial system as *gripping*. These gripping types of strategy generally occur in the presence of an imbalance between the deep and superficial myofascial systems, where there is inhibition of the deep system and over-activation of the superficial system as a means of increasing stability somewhere within our body.

Gripping

Gripping as a stabilization strategy has become so ubiquitous that we have come to think of these strategies as normal. Even some of the common cues used in the fitness industry—such as "pull in your abdominals" or "squeeze your shoulder blades down and back" or "tighten your tush"—can actually encourage these gripping strategies, because they are so effective at facilitating the use of the superficial myosfascial system.

Do Not Make a Habit of Gripping

A gripping strategy—an over-activation of the superficial myofascial system—is an effective compensatory stabilization strategy for inhibition of the deep myofascial system. This strategy is effective because it protects us against sudden loading or changes of force on our joints. However, the strategy is problematic when it becomes our habitual strategy, because it can lead to increased compression on the joints, myofascial tension, and restricted range of motion. Thus it is imperative to improve function of the deep myofascial system and institute an integrative movement strategy designed to restore balance between the deep and superficial systems.

Gripping syndromes are a major reason why so many of us experience chronic tightness, despite our attempts to mitigate it with foam rolling, stretching, and/or massage. We are generally over-contracting our muscles to a greater degree than we should in order to perform simple tasks such as standing, walking, or activities of daily life; moreover, we do not let these muscles relax when we no longer have need of them. In other words, we are over-recruiting our superficial myofascial system to compensate for inhibition of the deeper system.

For example, when performing Leg Circles, Teaser, and Side-Lying Leg Circles, you first activate the deep myofascial system—primarily the psoas and deep hip rotators—to align and center (centrate) the femoral head within the acetabulum and activate the diaphragm, pelvic floor, transversus abdominis, multifidi, and other deep spinal stabilizers to stabilize the spine and pelvis. Next, you will activate the superficial muscles of the hip (rectus femoris, tensor fasciae latae, adductors, and hamstrings) to move the hip, and the superficial abdominals and erector spinae muscles to help stabilize the spine and pelvis against the potential movement that occurs because the legs are moving.

Now suppose your deep myofascial system is inhibited or you have over-activated your superficial myofascial system by performing too many repetitions as you fatigued, and you soldiered on with less than optimal hip centering and alignment. As the joint becomes increasingly misaligned throughout the current and subsequent workouts, the nervous system reacts by tightening the muscles around the joint (primarily the superficial myofascial system) to create better stabilization. However, you are now also using these superficial muscles as part of your daily routine, involving activities such as standing and walking. Over-activation of these muscles is becoming a habit. You may begin to notice tightness in the superficial muscles when you are sitting at home at night, a time when they should be relaxing. The more active you become walking, running, biking, doing Pilates, etc., the more ingrained this overuse pattern becomes.

To disrupt these habitual patterns of over-activity or gripping, we must first improve our motor control, or the way in which our nervous system is initiating and controlling posture and movement. Often we have to scale back the intensity of our exercise patterns so that we can relax the superficial system and activate our deep myofascial system.

Using the example of Leg Circles, let's look at how we can improve activation of the deep myofascial system and coordinate its use with the superficial system. To improve performance of the hip circle, we will use lying hip flexion with core activation (activation of the transversus abdominis and pelvic floor with diaphragmatic breathing) to optimize connection to the deep myofascial system while inhibiting the gripping of the superficial system.

To improve hip centration during her functional activities, the woman in Figure 5.9 is performing three-dimensional breathing and coordinating it with activation of her deep myofascial system. She then palpates the region of excessive gripping—usually the rectus femoris, tensor fasciae latae, or adductors—to make sure it stays relatively relaxed throughout the pattern. She visualizes a wire connecting from her spine just above her belly button to deep inside her hip, and begins to draw her leg into the socket, making the connection between her spine and hip. She ensures that the superficial hip flexors stay relaxed during this pattern, because she is working on developing the motor control to move her hip without gripping to flex her hip by excessively using the superficial myofascial system. After she can activate the deep system without compensatory gripping of the superficial system, she is taught how to incorporate this strategy into higher-level patterns.

By performing Leg Circles with her feet in straps to help unweight the leg, she can visualize sinking the hip into the socket as she performs the patterns. Once she has developed the motor control, she can progress to other high-level patterns, being mindful to not over-grip her superficial hip flexors.

Increase Awareness of Gripping
It is important to bring a client's awareness to where they are gripping, so that they can both feel and monitor it themselves. Teaching them how to palpate the region of over-activity, or gripping, is an important step in helping them relax and let go during the corrective exercise process.

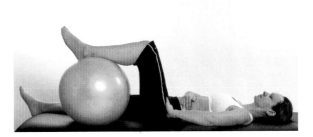

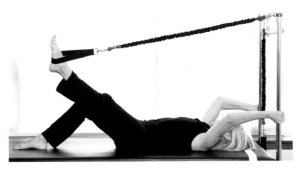

Figure 5.9: Coordination of three-dimensional breathing and activation of the deep myofascial system.

With optimal control, you do not feel the need to grip for stabilization or movement. The deep and superficial myofascial systems are balanced and react accordingly without gripping, unless gripping is specifically required for the task in hand. The key to improving function is to develop an efficient core stabilization strategy so that you do not have to resort to a gripping strategy to make up for the lack of joint control.

However, when you lose the ability to maintain an efficient core stabilization strategy, gripping becomes the primary compensatory strategy. The three main regions of gripping that directly affect core function are the back, abdominals, and hips. The particular strategy adopted by an individual will vary based on their neurodevelopment, history of trauma and surgery, exercise selection, and all the additional factors we have considered in the previous chapter.

Back Gripping

Individuals who are back grippers tend to develop hypertonicity around the region of the spine where contraction is the greatest. Although it can occur in any area of the spine, back gripping is common around the thoracolumbar region. There will generally be an increase in the thoracolumbar lordotic curvature, which will be associated with a decreased range of motion of flexion in this region. The body will compensate for this by segmentally flexing around the area of hypertonicity or the over-compressed region. This level of segmental flexion, or what we commonly refer to as *flexion instability*, is a part of the spine that is more mobile in flexion than it should be or is excessively flexed because the surrounding spinal segments have been over-compressed into extension: in other words, it is that area where the individual compensates (in this case by flexion) in order to create motion. This region of flexion becomes an area of instability that often leads to lumbar disc problems and/or nerve-related pain.

Note the hypertonicity in the lower to mid-thoracic spine, the compensatory thoracolumbar extension, and the flexion instability in the lumbar spine (the "bump" that seems to be sticking out of the back) in both of the patients shown in Figure 5.10. This region of flexion generally occurs as a result of the tightness and gripping above it. The client will usually experience pain and dysfunction here because they are not controlling that spinal segment, thereby causing irritation of the discs, nerves, and soft tissues of that region.

As we have mentioned, gripping can occur anywhere along the spine. Recall the earlier patient we presented with the lordosis from her lumbar spine through her thoracic spine. She presented with upper thoracic erector gripping

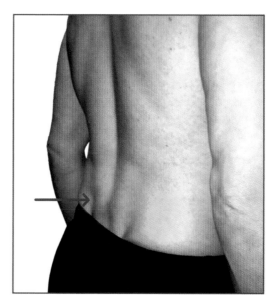

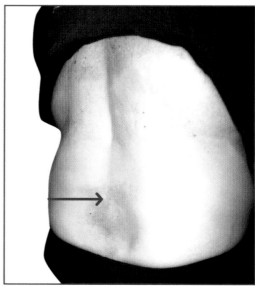

Figure 5.10: Spinal flexion as a result of tightness and gripping.

along with chronic headaches and right shoulder tightness. Note the lordosis through her entire spine: this limited her ability to fully utilize the posterior aspect of her diaphragm or to open up her thorax posteriorly, causing her to overuse her accessory breathing muscles (the scalenes, SCM, and pectoralis minor), resulting in a forward-head position and the chronic headaches. Once we got her to focus on releasing her over-contracted erectors and breathing into her back, she was able to release the chronic tension in her neck and significantly reduce the frequency and severity of her headaches.

Back gripping can be exacerbated by exercises such as hyperextensions or Swimming, because the individual continues to overwork an already over-contracted group of muscles. Back grippers tend to have high levels of resting tone in their erector spinae muscles, and these types of extension-biased exercise can perpetuate the use of the erectors in the role of extension.

As mentioned, gripping can occur as a result of some common cues we give our clients. Cues such as "lift your chest" and "squeeze your shoulder blades down and back," in particular, can lead to back gripping: a combination of these two actions will often cause an individual to grip through their shoulders and back, which will inhibit breathing and proper shoulder function.

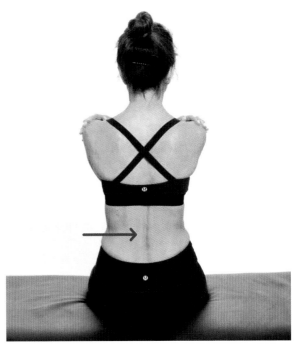

Figure 5.11: Resting tone in a client's lumbar erectors just when sitting quietly.

Figure 5.11 shows one of our clients who was taught these same cues in gymnastics from the time she was a little girl. Notice the amount of resting tone in her lumbar erectors just in quiet sitting. Palpation of these muscles confirmed that there was a high level of tone present, but this level of myofascial tone in these superficial muscles is not required, or desired, for a task like quiet sitting. This is another reason why so many of our clients experience back problems with sitting: they do not relax their muscles, so they are virtually sitting in a state of erector spinae contraction all day long.

Recall our earlier discussions about the studies conducted on individuals with chronic low back pain. Remember, these individuals not only used a stiffening or bracing stabilization strategy, but were also unable to turn their muscles off after a sudden perturbation (sudden change in their center of gravity), compared with the individuals without back pain. This emphasizes that knowing how to relax or turn our muscles off when they are not needed is just as important as knowing how to activate and turn the *right* muscles on. Using the right muscles when needed, and not overusing but rather relaxing them when not needed, are important parts of motor control training, and this strategy will be one of our goals throughout the corrective exercise and progressive exercise patterns.

What does this back gripping look like functionally? Another patient we introduced earlier with low back pain is shown in Figure 5.12. He experienced pain while standing and walking, but not while he was sitting or when he was playing soccer, which he did once a week. Notice the significant hypertonicity of his thoracolumbar erector spinae muscles. What is interesting is that this individual has never lifted weights in his life and he sits for work; so why are these muscles so developed?

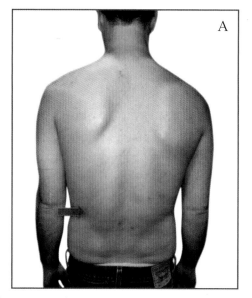
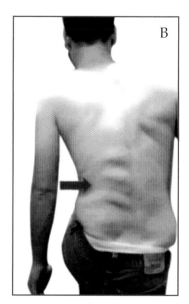

Figure 5.12: (a) A patient with low back pain; (b) single-leg stance test for this patient.

Looking at his single-leg stance test (Figure 5.11(b)), we see exactly why he has more problems in standing and walking. Note the significant increase in hypertonicity as he balances on one leg. Because of his poor breathing and core stabilization strategy (i.e., inhibition of the deep myofascial system), he overuses his superficial myofascial system— primarily the erector spinae muscles—for trunk stability in the single-leg stance. This is a common strategy for many of us, especially those who experience chronic hypertonicity and/or trigger points in our erector spinae muscles and/or quadratus lumborum.

Abdominal Gripping

The next area where over-contraction of the superficial myofascial system is frequently found is the abdominals (Figure 5.12). Abdominal gripping is very common, even among people who appear quite fit because they have been taught and/or have taught themselves to walk around with a contracted abdomen. While this may look aesthetically pleasing (making the waistline appear smaller), the response of the body in the long term to this gripping strategy is not favorable.

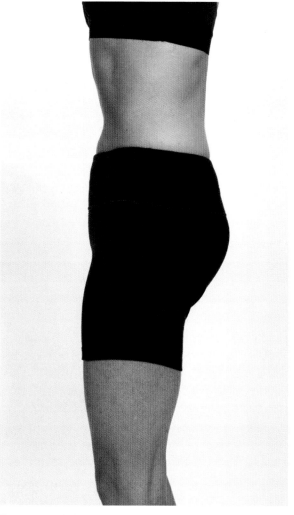

Figure 5.13. Abdominal gripping.

To get a sense of why gripping is not a good long-term strategy for stabilization, try the following experiment. As you sit there reading this book, contract the biceps of one arm and maintain this contraction as you read the next couple of pages. Now imagine what would happen if you walked around with your biceps contracted like this all day long. Within a few days this muscle would be hypertonic and fatigued, and your elbow would likely feel stiff and achy. The same thing is true for the abdominal muscles, as well as for the joints around your ribcage and spine, when you walk around with a contracted, or gripped, abdominal wall. Since the abdominals pull on your ribcage and pelvis, they compress your low back, in a similar way that contracting your biceps compressed your elbow. As with the elbow demonstration, over time this gripping strategy irritates the ligaments, discs, and joints of the spine.

Similarly to back gripping, abdominal gripping also occurs as a direct result of many of the cues we have been given in exercise classes, magazines, and other fitness-related media outlets. Cues like "pull your abs in," "brace your core," "tighten your stomach like you're going to get punched," and "tighten your tummy" are just a few of the common cues we have adopted in the fitness industry. There are three key reasons why we do not advocate them:

1. While we touched on this briefly in an earlier section, there are several problems associated with using a prolonged abdominal gripping strategy. A high level of abdominal tone increases the compressive forces on the system, especially when there is subsequent co-activation of the lumbar erectors to help control the flexion force placed on the spine. This leads to increased compression on the system from the co-activation of both the abdominals and the erectors. Just as we

demonstrated with the biceps earlier, over time the joints of your spine, pelvis, and hips will not respond well to prolonged compression.

2. Excessive and perpetual gripping of the abdominal region does not allow the individual to properly use the diaphragm, since its movement will be restricted in the TPC. This compromises respiration and thus inhibits decompression of the spine, since the individual will not be able to optimally utilize intra-abdominal pressure to stabilize their spine. This, in turn, leads to increased abdominal pressure moving down into the pelvic cavity; over time the pelvic floor becomes unable to match the pressure coming from above, since either it is not being reflexively activated by a properly functioning diaphragm, or there is simply too much downward pressure. Often this results in pelvic floor dysfunction and urinary incontinence.

3. Although we have a few clients and patients who have difficulty tightening or pulling in their abdominal wall, bracing the abdominal wall, for the majority, becomes their default strategy for stabilizing their core, especially after abdominal surgery and with chronic GI irritation. If our patients or clients do not have a problem performing these abdominal "draw-in" strategies, then it does not make sense to continue to use that strategy to improve core function. If something is relatively easy to do, it generally means that the individual does not need to continue to train that strategy. For these clients, we strive to develop a more efficient strategy that encourages the transversus abdominis, along with the rest of the deep myofascial system, to activate and develop a low level of tension without increasing the abdominal gripping that can result from an overeager interpretation of "tighten your tummy." A

surprising number of people are efficient at over-recruiting the superficial myofascial system (oblique abdominals and rectus abdominis) to draw their abdominals in. Remember that walking around with a gripped abdominal wall is no better than walking around with your arms flexed all day.

You can modify the cues you use to improve deep abdominal wall and pelvic floor co-activation by experimenting with a few of the options given in Table 5.1.

Common Cues	Modify with These Phrases
Tighten your tummy	… using only 10% of your strength.
Pull your abs in	… gently, like a soft vacuum seal, towards the spine.
Scoop your abs	… from the bottom up. Imagine a net lifting your internal organs, just an inch or so, from the pubic bone towards the ribcage.
Brace your core	… from deep within, at the level of the spinal bones, or in the light and quick manner you would if you stepped waist-deep into a cold lake.

Table 5.1: Cueing abdominal contraction without encouraging gripping.

Recall Evan's patient who had a cesarean section and GI resection (Chapter 4). She is attempting to provide additional support for the muscle inhibition that occurred as a result of these surgeries and hence lives with her belly pulled in. In order to develop improved strategies that do not rely exclusively on gripping, we need to learn to release the over-contraction, decrease the chronic tension in our abdominal muscles, and promote flexibility within the TPC. This supports a more efficient breathing strategy and decreases pressure on the spine through the development of intra-abdominal pressure.

Additionally, optimal three-dimensional breathing enables the diaphragm to push down and essentially massage our viscera, thereby improving abdominal circulation, which will improve the function of our entire body. Releasing chronic gripping can dramatically impact our entire system, because it supports mobility of the soft tissue as well as of blood and lymph tissue.

The patient in Figure 5.14 is another example of an abdominal gripper; note the loss of lumbar lordosis and posterior pelvic tilt. Such an individual can be a challenge to improve, since his chronic gripping has led to a shortening of the abdominal wall. The combination of performing 100 crunches a day for many years and then sitting at his job for the past 35 years of his life has resulted in increased thoracic kyphosis, posterior pelvic tilt, and lumbar spine flexion. As a consequence of this strategy, he experiences low back pain and sciatica. He was taught to release his abdominal wall and develop more control of a neutral spine and pelvic posture, which improved his posture and reduced his symptoms.

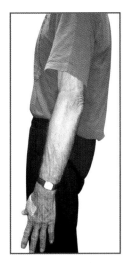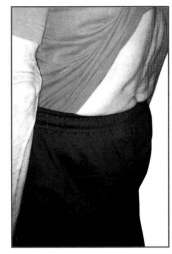

Figure 5.14: Another example of an abdominal gripper.

Individuals who grip their abdominals may struggle with training in a neutral spine position, but can be very effective at achieving the "flat back," or imprinted, spine position. The rectus abdominis and external obliques are capable of holding this position of the spine and pelvis, and can do so quite easily, even without the assistance of the deep myofascial system.

There is still some debate in the Pilates community about if and when an imprinted spine position should be used. The answer is: it depends. Some clients (such as those with spinal stenosis or spondylolisthesis) need to use extreme caution when attempting to achieve a neutral spine position, as it can cause irritation. For the vast majority of us who are not modern dancers or gymnasts (and especially anyone with disc herniations), we would be best advised to avoid the imprinted position altogether. The basic reasoning is that a flexed lumbar spine position places the most pressure on the discs of the low back. For this reason, to the extent that it is possible for the individual, we want to train the ability to recognize neutral spine as "home base," as this is the position in which the spine and discs are most protected. That said, lumbar flexion is a natural part of life, such as in forward bending and other daily activities. If you do incorporate an imprinted spine position as part of your practice, consider these prerequisites: correct breathing, proper activation of the deep myofascial system, and freedom from spinal complaints, such as disc problems or low back pain.

Training Neutral Pelvis in a Seated Position
For the person with a posteriorly tucked pelvis, the Stomach Massage exercise (Figure 5.15) is an ideal way to practice stabilizing the hips in a neutral position while stretching the posterior leg muscles responsible for pulling the pelvis out of position. It is also a great way for everyone to learn axial elongation. The discerning teacher will be able to cue, through touch, the exact spinal segments where lift is most compromised. These segments move more during the exercise, and the spinous process often feels more prominent to the touch. For a more forgiving variation of Stomach Massage, reduce the springs to one and lower the feet to the lower sides of the footbar or the platform.

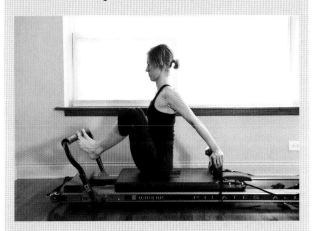

Figure 5.15: Stomach Massage exercise.

An exercise from Shirley Sahrmann is another excellent way to correct the posteriorly tucked pelvis pattern, and can be incorporated into the Short Box routine. Remove one foot from under the safety strap and hold it under the thigh. Sitting up tall, pelvis in neutral, practice lengthening and bending the leg while maintaining a long spine. Like Stomach Massage, this will challenge you to anchor your pelvis and low back against the powerful tug of your hamstrings. Then try letting go of the leg and holding it up a few inches off the ground while you maintain a long spine. For an additional challenge, press down into the top of the leg as the leg presses up into the palms of your hands. Continue to elongate the low spine against the compressive force of your hip flexor contracting.

Hip Gripping

While technically not part of the TPC, the hip complex will directly impact the alignment and function of the pelvis and lumbar spine. When there is an optimal balance between the deep and superficial myofascial systems, the femoral head remains relatively centered in the acetabulum during most functional activities (Figure 5.16(a)); likewise, the pelvis remains supported and controlled around the femoral heads.

However, when the posterior and/or lateral hip muscles are over-contracted (gripping), they can disrupt the optimal alignment of the femoral head within the acetabulum and drive the femoral head forward (Figure 5.16(b)). This disrupts the axis of hip rotation during functional activity and creates wear and tear across the anterior and superior portions of the femoral head. Additionally, this gripping alters the position and control of the pelvis over the top of the femoral heads and leads to many of the postural changes we see,

including anterior or posterior rotation and lateral tilting of the pelvis; it even contributes to leg-length discrepancies.

We believe that this anterior femoral head position directly leads to many of the common issues we are seeing in our patients and clients, including femoroacetabular impingement (FAI), labral tears (tearing of the labrum around the acetabulum as a result of the forward femoral head position), and long-term degenerative changes.

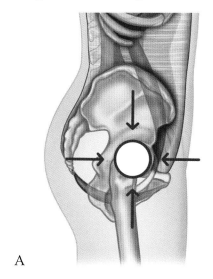

A

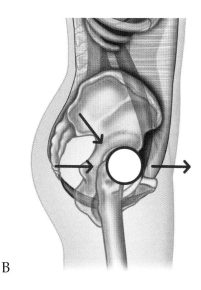

B

Figure 5.16: (a) Centrated hip; (b) anterior femoral head position.

Hip gripping is characterized by an over-contraction of the posterior and/or lateral hip complex and is indicated by a hollowing, or "divot," that can be palpated in the lateral thigh region, just superior to and behind the greater trochanter. If the gripping has been a long-term strategy, generally some wasting of the lower medial fibers of the gluteus maximus has occurred, as demonstrated by the patient in Figure 5.17, who presented with over-activation of the superficial fibers of the gluteus maximus and some of the deeper hip rotators.

The client in Figure 5.17 is a classic example of a hip gripper. Note the indentation, or hollowing, in his lateral hips caused by the contraction of his posterior and lateral hip muscles as a result of over-activating his hips during his lower body exercise patterns, such as squats, lunges, and step-ups. Because of this hip-gripping strategy he lives in a perpetual state of chronic tightness, which could eventually lead to a labral tear of his hip.

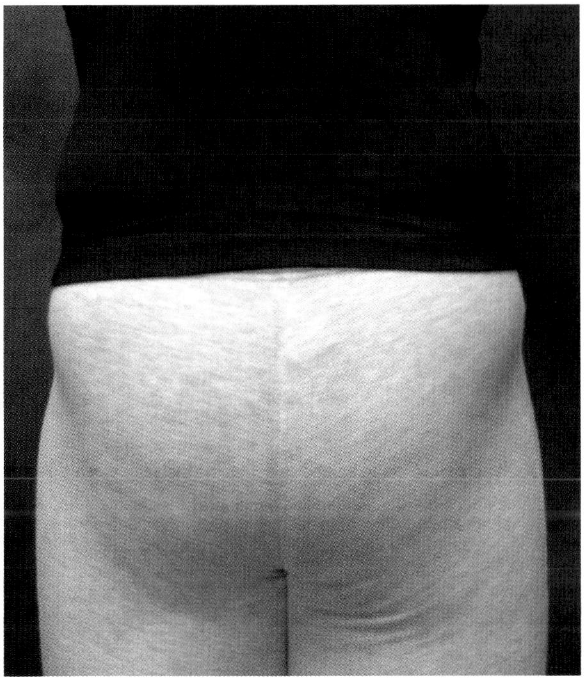

Someone can be a hip gripper even without the signs of lateral divots. These individuals generally present with increased resting hypertonicity of the superficial glutes, hip abductors/adductors, and/or hip flexors and restriction in their hip range of motion. If you are a hip gripper and are able to maintain a relatively optimal position for hip motion, you will still over-compress the femoral head into the acetabulum and over time increase wear and tear on the soft tissue and bony structure of the hip.

How does hip gripping manifest during functional activities? It is best seen when the individual flexes or rotates their pelvis or hips. Hip grippers generally lose the ability to move optimally through their hips and have to compensate by preferentially moving through the knees or low back when squatting or bending forward. This increases stress on the low back and/or knees to compensate for the lack of hip motion.

Figure 5.17: A classic example of a hip gripper.

Figure 5.18 shows a professional athlete who presented with chronic low back discomfort, not significant enough to keep him from playing, but enough to affect his performance during exercise and practice. Upon evaluation, it was found that he had significant posterior and lateral hip gripping, and hypertonicity in his thoracolumbar erector spinae muscles (see Figure 5.18). As he bends forward, note the lack of anterior pelvic tilt because of the posterior hip gripping, which he compensates for by over-flexing his lumbar spine. This region of increased movement is the exact location in which he experiences low back pain. The hip restriction forces him to sit in a posterior pelvic tilt and lumbar spine flexion, which will perpetuate core dysfunction.

The athlete in Figure 5.18 clearly demonstrates how these gripping strategies can lead to compensatory instability elsewhere in the kinetic chain. If we do not change these patterns we will be significantly limited in how much we can improve our stabilization and movement. Pilates reformer exercises—such as Elephant, Washer Woman variations on the chair (straight and rounded spine), or modified Stomach Massage (with footbar lowered or even sitting on the short box)—offer the perfect opportunity to retrain this pattern.

Note
It is sometimes necessary for taller people and those with tight posterior hips to sit on a bolster during short box and wunda chair exercises. As a general rule, when an individual with hip gripping is seated, the knees should not be higher than the hips, as this will pull the pelvis into a posterior tuck.

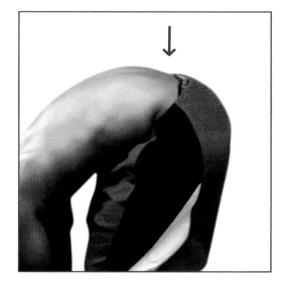

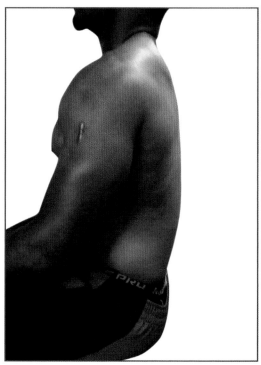

Figure 5.18: Professional athlete with chronic low back discomfort.

There are several other ways in which hip gripping manifests in our functional activities. Note the gentleman performing burpees during his group exercise class in Figure 5.19; how well does he flex his hips? He gets very little anterior pelvic tilt because he is over-gripping his posterior hip complex, so he has to compensate by over-flexing through his thoracic spine.

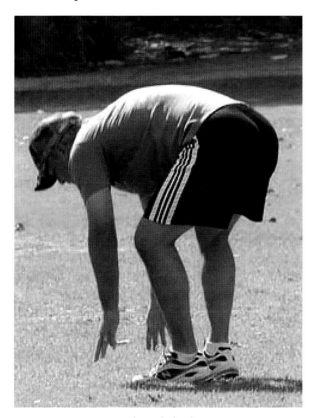

Figure 5.19: Over-flexing through the thoracic spine to compensate for over-gripping the posterior hip complex while performing burpees.

As the woman in Figure 5.20 performs a barbell squat, you will notice the increased thoracic extension and lumbar flexion as she nears the bottom position. During the squat pattern, when she runs out of hip flexion range of motion, she begins to posteriorly rotate her pelvis and flex even further through her lumbar spine. These are movement strategies that increase stress on both the low back and the sacroiliac joints, in addition to the hips.

We can also recognize this inability to move through the posterior and lateral hips during Pilates patterns. Training a neutral pelvis during Leg Springs is an ideal way to open up the hips in a safe, low-load environment. As we gain competence in stabilizing the pelvis in neutral, the hips become more flexible and we achieve greater ease and functional range of motion in this exercise. Lunge Variations on the Reformer, Standing One-Leg Press on the Chair, and Going Up Front on the Chair offer additional opportunities to strengthen and reinforce this kinesthetic awareness in standing.

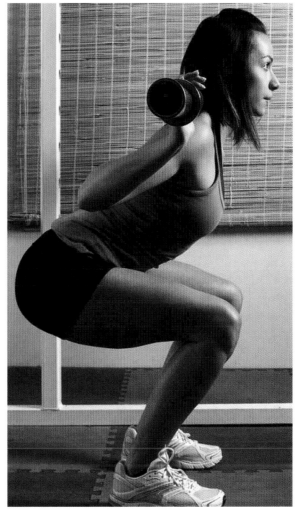

Figure 5.20: Posterior rotation of the pelvis and increased flexion of the lumbar spine near the end position of a barbell squat.

Hip Gripping During Footwork and Leg Springs

Gripping the hips during Footwork and Leg Springs can be seen as tucking the pelvis, especially during the initiation of hip and knee extension. The lower fibers of the glutes are drawn in and the pelvis may jump a bit off the carriage as the legs begin to straighten against the weight of the springs. Once you point it out to them, most people can recognize that they are, in fact, gripping. If they cannot recognize it, you might ask them to squeeze their bottom as tight as they can, and then relax it. Suggest that they imagine the feeling as if they were to pass gas (and, if appropriate, encourage them that it is okay if they do). It is absolutely necessary to create a supportive and professional environment, particularly when asking clients to concentrate on their pelvic floor muscles.

Standing One-Leg Press on the Chair

Those with exceptionally tight posterior hips will succumb to a tuck in the pelvis as the pedal rises. You might also notice their torso shifting back in response to this movement. Recognizing this tendency is the first step in correcting it. Limit the upward range of the pedal and always elongate the spine.

Why take the time to correct hip-gripping patterns? With chronic hip gripping, we are unable to fully relax the body at rest, which perpetuates hypertonicity, trigger points, and muscle fatigue as well as many of our chronic musculoskeletal problems.

There is another plausible explanation why so many individuals grip their hips. We believe that many hip-gripping cases not only stem from habitual patterns, but are also a reaction by the nervous system to help support the pelvic floor. In discussions with Dr. Judy Florendo, a physical therapist specializing on the pelvic floor, she seems to agree with this theory.

So why does the pelvic floor need additional support when hip gripping occurs? Recall that when TPC stability is compromised and the individual is using a bracing or gripping strategy for control, there is a significant amount of inferiorly directed pressure in the abdominal and pelvic cavities. This is especially true when the individual has a stereotypical non-optimal breathing pattern and thus a poor ability to control intra-abdominal pressure. If the person is unable to use their diaphragm and transversus abdominis appropriately, they cannot generate intra-abdominal pressure and reflexively activate the pelvic floor; this leads to a greater tendency towards urinary incontinence as a result of this increased pressure. Although it is non-optimal, posterior hip gripping is an effective strategy for using the posterior hip muscles to aid pelvic floor support.

Many women experience stress incontinence (when coughing, sneezing, laughing, exercising), and for 30 percent of young female athletes, stress incontinence is an issue. How many individuals experience pelvic floor dysfunction, even if they are not actually leaking? If we are not breathing correctly, are overusing an accessory breathing strategy, or have inhibition of our deep myofascial system, it is probable that we lack the reflexive activation of the pelvis and that increased pressure is being placed upon it. Improving alignment, breathing, and activation of the deep myofascial system is an effective strategy for releasing chronic hip gripping and subsequent tightness.

Similarly to the other gripping patterns, many of the cues we have been taught throughout the fitness industry have helped perpetuate this dysfunction. Cues such as "tighten your tush," "squeeze your glutes," and "contract your backside" over-activate the posterior hip complex, which not only drives the femoral head forward within the acetabulum, but also rotates the pelvis into a posterior pelvic tilt.

Regarding posterior hip gripping, one question we continually ask ourselves is: do you have a difficult time squeezing our glutes? If you are similar to our clients and patients, then you do not have difficulty contracting or squeezing your glutes, either. Remember what we said earlier—if we can do something easily, we most likely do not need to be doing it, because it is probably already a part of our habitual strategy. Our goal is to improve the function of the glutes and integrate their function with the rest of the hip muscles to control the femoral head within the acetabulum as well as control the position of the pelvis.

Because we live in an aesthetics-driven culture, another common cause of hip gripping that warrants a mention is the over-contraction of the posterior or lateral hip complex in an attempt to improve the shape or tone of the hips. It is believed that squeezing or gripping the lower glutes will give us that desirable "butt lift." But does gripping actually improve the shape of our hips?

A well-shaped gluteal complex is roundish, or more like the shape of an upside-down heart (Figure 5.21(a)). With hip gripping, the individual will squeeze, contract, or grip with their superior gluteal fibers—those that insert into the iliotibial band and/or the deep rotators. Contraction of these fibers, in combination with the deep rotators, is responsible for driving the femoral head forward within the acetabulum.

Additionally this strategy alters the shape by contracting and squeezing the inferior gluteal region, making it nearly impossible for the individual to sit their femoral head back in their acetabulum or use their deeper, lower glutes (Figure 5.21(b)). As a result, the

individual will usually develop atrophy of the deeper lower and medial fibers of the glutes— the portion responsible for drawing the femoral head back in the acetabulum. So, not only does the shape of the glutes worsen as a result of this gripping, but the individual will also develop dysfunction of the hips, pelvis, and low back.

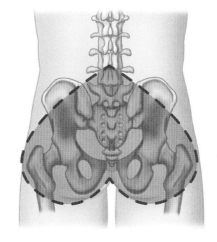

A

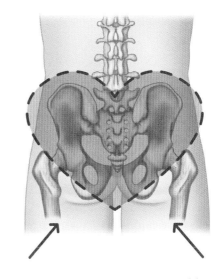

B

Figure 5.21: (a) A well-shaped gluteal complex. (b) Contracting and squeezing the inferior gluteal region makes it impossible for an individual to sit their femoral head back in their acetabulum or use their deeper, lower glutes.

A Great Way to Release Gripping Patterns in the Body: Learn to Shake your Tush!

If you want to learn how to loosen up the hips, abs, psoas, and low back, you can always take up a form of Latin dance (such as salsa or merengue), Brazilian dance, African dance, or belly dance. There is no way you can move like that without letting go of your hips! Dancing like this is a great way to help restore mobility, strength, and function to the hips and core. Remember, being present and mindful of your body's sensations is key to correcting faulty movement patterns. Put your brain on alert "learning" mode and let the Pilates principles guide you.

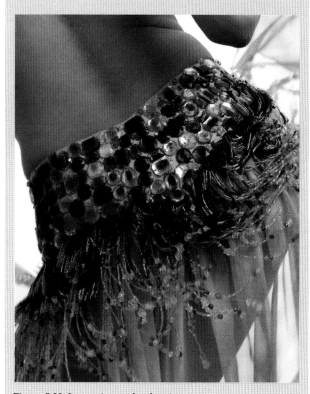

Figure 5.22: Loosening up by dancing.

Short- and Long-Term Effects of Gripping Strategies

So far, we have identified gripping strategies in three common areas—back, abdominals, and hips—in response to non-optimal core stabilization. We have discussed some of the challenges that gripping presents, including: the effect on our ability to breathe three-dimensionally; the inability to achieve intra-abdominal pressure; and the compensatory movement patterns, such as over-flexing the lumbar spine to compensate for lack of thoracolumbar motion (as a result of back gripping) or for inadequate anterior pelvic tilt contribution in forward bending (as a result of hip gripping). In this final section we highlight a few of the typical short- and long-term effects of these gripping strategies and talk about how they manifest in many of our common musculoskeletal syndromes.

Effects of Back and/or Abdominal Gripping

Recall that with back gripping, there will be a region of instability or hypermobility usually below the area of restriction. In the early stages of this instability, the individual may experience disc bulges and herniations (Figure 5.23). If this strategy continues, in an attempt to make the spine more stable the body will begin to lay down more bone: this is what medical doctors will label as *degenerative joint disease* or *osteoarthritis*. Over time, this bony growth will lead to stenosis—a narrowing of the spinal canal or foramina where the nerve roots exit the spinal canal—and other joint problems of the spine. While the medical profession will often blame the person's age or just label the degenerative changes as "normal," most of these changes are a direct result of our habitual patterns. In other words, we have created non-optimal stabilization strategies and movement patterns that have manifested as changes in soft tissue and bone.

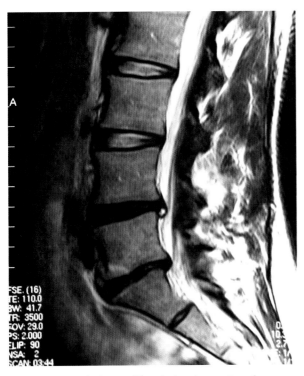

Figure 5.23: Disc bulges and herniations in a region of instability caused by hip gripping.

Effects of Hip Gripping

In the early stages of hip gripping, the individual will generally feel a sense of hip tightness or of always needing to foam roll or release the hip muscles. In general, the anterior position of the femoral head will not be felt within the acetabulum unless the individual has seen a qualified health practitioner who has been trained in palpating this position.

One of the first signs and symptoms the individual will experience, aside from tight hips, is FAI, which manifests as anterior and medial hip or groin pain when they flex, adduct, and internally rotate their hip (Figure 5.24). The impingement tends to occur during posterior hip stretches, with the leg pulled into flexion and adduction, or in deep squat positions with a narrow stance; essentially it occurs with any exercise that reproduces the hip-impingement position. Also associated with FAI, a forward position of the femoral head can lead to groin and adductor strains as well.

Get Rid of Hip Clicking

It is common for people to experience audible hip clicking during Leg Circles in the Pilates repertoire. Often clients find relief by connecting more deeply in their core and adding their own imaginary resistance to the hip-extension phase of the movement. In our experience, performing the movement by first activating the deep myofascial system and placing the involved-side foot in a leg spring or resistance band to take the weight off the leg (or reducing the lever by bending the knee) almost always eliminates the clicking.

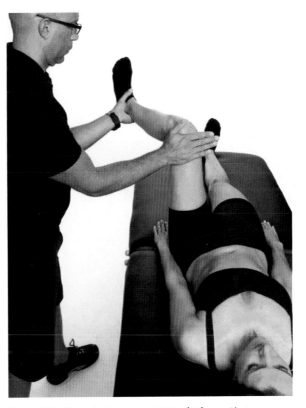

Figure 5.24: Hip gripping causes FAI, which manifests as anterior and medial hip or groin pain when flexing, adducting, and internally rotating the hip.

If pain and dysfunction persist and the individual continues to function with an anteriorly positioned hip, a labral tear of the hip can develop. This is an increasingly common injury in the athletic population, and we strongly believe that a major cause of these tears is non-optimal core and hip stabilization strategies that include over-gripping and increasing pressure down into the pelvis, followed by over-gripping of the posterior and lateral hip muscles to enhance hip stability.

The most significant long-term effects of hip gripping arise from the activity we tend to do the most during the day—sitting. When we over-grip our hips, we are unable to optimally position our pelvis over the top of the femoral heads; in other words, we cannot achieve a neutral pelvic position. When we cannot position our pelvis optimally, then we cannot properly align the spine over the pelvis. As a consequence, we tend to sit in a posterior pelvic tilt, with the weight of the trunk falling behind the pelvis; this increases the compressive forces into the low back, which overstretches the ligaments and soft tissue (creep). This affects our ability to do flexion-based activities or exercises without compromising the integrity of the spine and is one of the most common causes of disc injury and low back pain.

If a hip-gripping strategy continues for 20–30 years, there will be long-term effects from the dysfunctional stabilization and movement strategies. In X-ray images, there is usually a noticeable decrease in hip-joint space and increase in bony density around the hip (see Evan's patient in Figure 5.25). These individuals generally have significant discomfort, atrophy of the deep lower glutes, and hypertrophy of the superficial glutes.

These findings correspond with the research on individuals with degenerative hips, the results of which indicate that there tends to be atrophy of the deep myofascial system and hypertrophy of the superficial myofascial system of the hip (Grimaldi 2009).

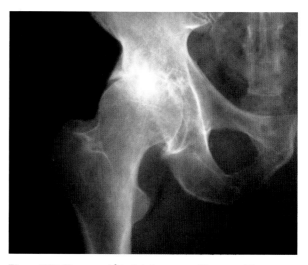

Figure 5.25: Decreased hip-joint space and increased bone density around the hip are long-term effects arising from a hip-gripping strategy.

When the medical history was being taken, Evan's patient reported that she had had one child delivered via cesarean section. Evan explained to her that this was probably the reason why she developed altered stabilization issues in her trunk and hip, and she mentioned that she did have back pain for at least one year after her delivery. This is a common sequence in the development of hip degeneration: abdominal or pelvic surgery ⋯→ non-optimal core stabilization strategies ⋯→ years of compensated movement strategies, including over-gripping from the hips ⋯→ and finally joint degeneration (Figure 5.26). The majority of these individuals can, however, benefit from an improved stabilization and movement strategy even after they have developed significant issues or after returning from surgery.

Conclusion

In this chapter we have looked at how the nervous system responds to non-optimal levels of core control created by muscle inhibition. A common nervous system strategy is to up-regulate, or over-contract (grip), throughout certain key regions of the trunk (erector spinae muscles and/or abdominals) or hips (primarily posterior and lateral hip musculature). These gripping strategies directly impact both our posture and how we perform daily activities (such as sitting), squatting, and Pilates exercises.

The important point is that many of our chronic myofascial tightness and pain manifestations as well as degenerative changes are the direct result of our habitual stabilization and movement patterns. Without addressing the imbalance between the deep and superficial myofascial systems, it is difficult, and often impossible, to change or improve how we stabilize and move. Often we must first relax or decrease myofascial over-activity (the individual's gripping strategy). Then we have to retrain our nervous system so that it chooses to preferentially recruit the deep myofascial system to develop the specific level of stabilization required by the joints. At that point, we can add the next layer—the superficial myofascial system—so that we can further stabilize and/or move to accomplish the desired task. This strategy has been discussed in part in earlier sections on breathing and core activation; we will now expand on this concept in the next chapter.

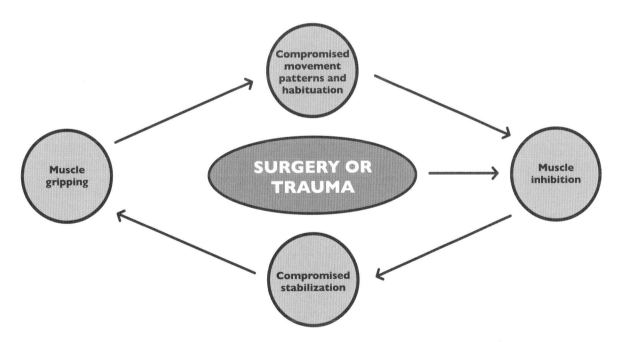

Figure 5.26: Muscle inhibition, a direct result of surgery or other trauma for example, compromises core stabilization. The nervous system reacts by over-activating, or gripping, which leads to a self-perpetuating cycle of compromised posture and movement.

Integrating the Pilates Principles

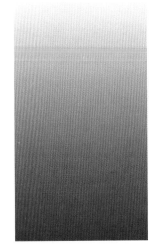

6

Every one of us has a physical history that has been shaped by lifestyle and environmental factors, traumatic events (such as surgeries or injuries), and neurodevelopmental challenges. Fitness trainers, including Pilates instructors, need to familiarize themselves with individual movement habits, especially those that may predispose someone toward pain or injury. By learning to recognize insidious patterns—such as chronic muscle gripping, abdominal bulging, pelvic imbalance, and faulty breathing—we can ensure that the exercise programs we implement are safe, appropriate, and beneficial over time.

Fortunately, the body and brain are designed for adaptation and change. Pilates exercises, when informed by the original six principles, are a wonderful way to restore functional balance and ease to the way we move (see Table 6.1).

In this chapter, we will look at how to apply everything we have covered thus far in this book to our practice of Pilates.

Pilates Principle	Lessons for Our Practice
Centering is about developing integral strength.	Seek to replace gripping or bracing patterns with deep core strength.
Concentration conveys that our state of mind makes a difference.	Stay attentive during workouts. Do not "check out."
Breath teaches that focusing and optimizing the breath is essential.	Make the breath a focal point of fitness practice. Pilates is a perfect opportunity to optimize breathing patterns.
Control aspires to a complete kinesthetic awakening and total mastery of the body.	The potential for awareness and mastery of the human body is endless. Keep an open mind.
Precision demands that we notice faulty habits; we tend to need subtle cues in order to overcome them.	Move slowly. Understand exactly what you are trying to do. Include basic patterns and lighter loads. There are no shortcuts.
Flow invites a smooth and pleasurable coordination of movement.	Integrate and explore movement patterns in a smooth and kinesthetically alive manner.

Table 6.1: Lessons for each of the six principles of Pilates.

Kinesthetic Milestones for the Pilates Powerhouse

Pilates is built around a few fundamental movement patterns that are combined in an ever-changing environment where new challenges can always keep the student interested. In this way, the practice becomes more profound over time, as a new dimension to long-traversed movements is revealed.

In Pilates, every exercise serves a dual purpose: an assessment tool *and* a corrective exercise. An experienced instructor watches their client move and looks for telltale signs of muscle imbalances and core weakness, providing tactile and verbal suggestions based on what they observe. The assessment process is ongoing and dynamic—an integrated part of the workout. Over time, with clear cues and repetition of key movements, unconscious patterns become recognized and re-patterned into more stable and efficient ones, resulting in energy, longevity, and overall well-being.

The Pilates exercises provide the structure for the above process, but the *living* part of it is *kinesthesia*—the awareness of, and feeling for, how your body moves. With the right state of mind, Pilates helps the body wake up to itself, and when needed, the Pilates instructor can point the way. In order to notice where the body is less "awake" to itself, the instructor must learn to recognize certain patterns. The list of kinesthetic milestones below provides a new organizational framework for developing this body consciousness in the core.

Each of the kinesthetic patterns listed can be emphasized in almost any Pilates exercise, though we recommend that you work with a limited number of focal points, so as not to overwhelm yourself or your client. You will determine which areas to focus on once you see your client moving. The slower they move and the more basic the pattern, the more they will *feel* and you will *see*. Choose your "headline" areas for the session (the most relevant or apparent kinesthetic challenges) and emphasize these over and over in different exercises.

1. Noticing and Releasing Gripping Patterns

The most commonly observed gripping patterns of the core are:

- back (quadratus lumborum, superficial paraspinals);
- abdominal (rectus abdominis and obliques);
- hip (flexors: tensor fasciae latae, rectus femoris, psoas; glutes; adductors; pelvic floor muscles).

2. Functional Core Activation

Learn to functionally engage and coordinate the TPC (rectus abdominis, transversus abdominis, obliques, diaphragm, pelvic floor, psoas, deep paraspinals), with the ability to:

- recognize and isolate these muscles, and distinguish the deep and superficial layers of the core;
- pre-activate the deep core before all movements;
- activate core muscles concentrically/eccentrically (change in lumbar spine) and isometrically (no change in lumbar spine);
- activate core muscles in varying degrees of intensity, engaging the appropriate level of muscle engagement for the task in hand.

3. Neutral Pelvis

Learn to find and stabilize the pelvis in neutral (or a modified version of neutral that is appropriate for the client), with isometric contraction of abdominals and deep back muscles:

- during loaded and unloaded movements of the limbs and thoracic spine;
- in various planes of movement (transverse, sagittal, coronal);
- in various planes of gravity (seated/standing, prone, sideways, supine, inverted).

4. Breathing

Develop the ability to control and direct intra-abdominal pressure for various activities by:

- learning to soften and expand the abdomen on the inhale;
- learning to keep the abdomen gently contracted throughout the full breath cycle;
- learning to align the respiratory diaphragm and expand the ribcage (laterally and posterolaterally) to stabilize the thoracolumbar junction on the inhale;
- being able to maintain openness of the ribs during the entire breath cycle;
- keeping the throat (glottis) open and the breath continuous during exercise and strenuous activity.

5. Axial Elongation

Develop the kinesthetic sense for elongation of the spine around its central axis with pelvic and respiratory diaphragms in alignment. Maintaining elongation (overcoming compressive and shearing forces) on all lumbar vertebral joints (T12 through S1):

• during loaded and unloaded movements of the limbs and thoracic spine;
• in various planes of movement (transverse, sagittal, coronal);
• in various planes of gravity (seated/ standing, prone, sideways, supine, inverted).

6. Thoracic Mobility

Increase thoracic mobility and articulation in flexion, extension, rotation, lateral flexion, and combinations of these movements.

7. Flow

Learn to bring the right amount of co-ordinated effort to the exercise, and recognize and adjust for jerky, bulging, collapsing, or overly braced movements, including the ability to:

• recognize and adjust the source and intensity of movements as required;
• leverage the superficial myofascial chains for power and stability (acceleration and deceleration) of variable forces while leveraging tensile stability in the deep core;
• engage fascial recoil in plyometric activities;
• confidently and spontaneously negotiate both the expected and the unexpected in the physical environment, and doing so with pleasure and efficiency.

In practice, many of these milestones overlap and you will not teach them in isolation. As the function in one area improves, so will the function in another. For example:

• Learn to find and stabilize a neutral-pelvis position involves isometric abdominal contraction, axial elongation, and awareness of any gripping tendencies.

• Along with axial elongation, clients will begin to develop:
  o thoracic mobilization and costal–lateral breathing as they side bend and rotate with a long lumbar spine;
  o posterolateral breathing, as they learn to elongate the spine without hinging at the thoracolumbar junction;
  o awareness and relaxation of any gripping patterns.

• Both flow and an unrestricted and continuous breath will develop along the way as clients learn to bring the right amount of coordinated (deep and superficial) muscular effort to a movement.

Every single Pilates exercise offers an opportunity to teach these milestones, but learning will not necessarily happen without the right blend of intellectual understanding and kinesthetic awareness. Look, listen, palpate, and sense for these milestones in your own practice and in your clients'. Start slowly with lower-load exercises. Encourage curiosity about sensations and attention to nuance. This will help build the awareness needed to replace habitual patterns with more functional ones. A good rule of thumb for sessions is to allocate 20–30% to instruction in the form of precise and succinct cueing and allow 70–80% as space for the client to explore and develop kinesthetic awareness. Some helpful cues to bring awareness to these kinesthetic milestones are presented in the next section.

Cues to Build Kinesthetic Awareness

Gripping Pattern Release

- Abdominal: Gently massage the sides of your stomach with the heels of your hands and notice any sensations. Do you feel bloated or tight? Use your inhalations to coax space into your abdomen. Soften the belly and let it rise into your hands.

- Back: Gently massage the large muscles and surrounding tissues of your mid- to low back (you can use your hands or a foam roller). Notice the tension and encourage it to release.

- Glutes/Pelvic Floor: Notice if you are holding any extra tension in your bottom. If you are not sure, try squeezing your bottom as tight as you can and then completely relaxing it.
  - Visualize the pubic bone, sitz bones, and tailbone. They form a diamond-shaped frame for your pelvic floor muscles. Gently contract only the anterior portion by imagining you are trying to stop a stream of urine, and release. Gently contract only the posterior portion by imagining you are trying to stop yourself from passing gas, and release. Next gently lift the area in between (the vagina for women, the testicles for men), and release. Now connect all three points, imagining a hammock or a supportive harness lifting your organs.
  - Imagine bringing the sitz bones closer together without squeezing the glutes. Now imagine bringing the pubic bone and tailbone together without squeezing the glutes. (Advanced) Experiment with bringing the diagonal points together (e.g., left sitz bone to tailbone, right sitz bone to tailbone, left sitz bone to pubic bone, right sitz bone to pubic bone).

- Obliques: Place your hands on your low belly at an angle (as if they are in your pants pockets), with your pinky fingers resting just above the inguinal crease. Imagine your external obliques running in this direction. Notice any tension in this area and attempt to soften it. Now gently tone the muscles beneath your pinky fingers without clenching your glutes. Can you isolate one side and then the other? Carry this contraction towards your ring finger, your middle finger, etc. (obliques). Now try to relax these muscles completely and see if you can gently engage the abdominals *without* feeling the obliques "pop" up into the fingers.

- Hip flexor: Lie supine, with the legs propped on a stability ball or on the reformer footbar. Activate your deep core as described in the Functional Core Activation section below. With one hand, palpate the front of your hip to ensure that you are not gripping in the hip flexors or inner thighs. Visualize a deep wire connecting from the front of your spine to the front of your hip near the groin area (psoas muscle). Still activating the deep core, slowly slide your leg along the ball, or press out on the reformer, and then return to the start position. Lightly palpate the front of your hips and feel how the muscles activate as you move. Notice any difference left to right. See how it feels to bring less (or more) muscular energy to the movement. Don't concern yourself with right or wrong, necessarily. Just explore and allow your body to become aware of its options.

- Resolving excess myofascial tension is an essential part of rebuilding functional core strength. Your client may need to see a manual therapist and/or conduct self-care for chronic myofascial tension. An excellent resource for trigger point self-care is *The Trigger Point Therapy Workbook by Clair Davies* (2004).

Functional Core Activation

- First, you must soften the belly. Place your hands on your stomach. On the inhale, feel the belly gently rise into the palms of your hands. On the exhale, feel the tummy flesh gently pull away from the hands. (Once you have established awareness of breathing patterns and the ability to soften the belly, move on to the following cues.)

- Gently contract the low abdominals, starting at the pubic bone, and then, like slowly zipping up a zipper, continue this lift to the navel. Imagine an internal net or harness lifting your intestines gently towards your ribcage, releasing the downward pressure of all the organs on the pelvic floor.

- Imagine narrowing the waistline very softly, as if gently tightening a belt or drawing the hip bones towards one another (TVA).

Neutral Pelvis

- Lying supine, place your hand under your low back, maintaining a small back curve. Contract the abdominal muscles without pressing your back down into your hand.

- Make a triangle with your thumbs and pointer fingers. Place the heel of the hands on the bony hip bones (ASISs) and the fingertips on the pubic bone. The triangle should be parallel to the ceiling (or wall in front of you, if standing).

- To better feel the deep back muscles, gently contract the pelvic floor muscles (pubic bone to tailbone) without squeezing the glutes. Now, carry this sensation around the back of the tailbone to the posterior surface of the sacrum (the upside-down triangle-shaped bone at the back of the pelvis). Can you bring this same feeling into the deep bones of the low back? Sense a gentle tension in and around the low back bones.

Breathing

- Feel the lower ribs expand to the side like the handles of a bucket lifting up and down with each breath. Try holding the ribs open for a few seconds at a time, then release.

- Breathe volume into the band that wraps around from the base of the sternum to just below your shoulder blades. Keep this fullness on your exhale.

- Breathe into the space between the sternum and the heart. Imagine inflating a balloon all around your heart, with each breath coaxing a little more space into this area.

Axial Elongation

- Imagine that your spinal cord is made of rubber and elongate from the tailbone to the crown.

- (If you see hinging at the TLJ) Breathe into the back ribs and keep the ribs open as you exhale so that the ribcage aligns over the pelvis.

Thoracic Mobility

- A stuck or immobile area of the spine indicates that adjacent areas require more stability. Therefore, cue axial elongation through the entire spine, especially in the spinal segment(s) just below the area of restriction; then call for movement in the restricted area.

Flow

- Notice where your movement jerks, or "hiccups." Can you slow down through these parts of the movement and find a smoother, less effortful way to move?

- Everything flows from the core and reverberates back into it. Feel this inter-connection of all parts of the body as you move.

- Remember your milestones: elongate the spine, open the ribs, breathe, and move with grace and ease!

Identifying Areas of Kinesthetic Challenge

As mentioned before, every Pilates exercise is an assessment. Here are some examples of exercises that contain basic movement patterns and make it easy to identify areas of kinesthetic challenge for your client. Use verbal, visual (including imagery), and tactile cues to help them recognize proper alignment, release areas of gripping, lengthen and mobilize areas of tightness or compression, and discover new options they were not aware they had.

Kinesthetic Milestone	Pilates Exercises
Functional Core Activation Can the client bring the appropriate amount of deep core muscular engagement to basic movement patterns, such as …	• Supine Footwork? • Leg Springs? • Knee Stretch Variations? • Elephant? • Washer Woman on the Exo/Wunda Chair? • Roll-Down with Springs and Round Back on Short Box? • Standing One-Leg Press on the Chair?
Neutral Pelvis Can the client maintain neutral pelvis in …	• Supine Footwork? • Leg Circles on the Mat? • A crunch? • Seated hip flexion/extension patterns, including Stomach Massage variations and seated Footwork on the Wunda/Exo Chair? • Standing One-Leg Press on the Chair?
Breathing	Abdominal–Lumbar: • In supine, can the client fill their belly with air on inspiration and gently contract the abdominal muscles on expiration? • How about in Round Back Variations on the short box?

Kinesthetic Milestone	Pilates Exercises

Breathing (continued)	Posterolateral Breathing:
	• On inspiration, can the client expand the TLJ:
	  o In quadruped position and/or Child's Pose?
	  o During Bridging patterns on the mat or reformer?
	  o During seated Short Box Variations, such as arm raises with the pole, rotation, and Straight Spine Reach Back?
	  o Standing against a wall (challenge: with arms in goal post, as in Wall Angels)?
	• On exhalation, can the client maintain expansion of the TLJ?

Axial Elongation Can the client recognize and correct for unwanted compressive, flexion, and shearing forces on the individual vertebral segments during …	Mid-Thoracic/Sternal: • Can the client increase the volume in this area during standing and seated Roll-Down variations (against wall, Spine Stretch Forward, etc.)?
Gripping Patterns in Back, Abdominals, and Hips	• Short Box: lateral flexion, rotation, reach back? • Seated hip flexion/extension patterns, including Stomach Massage variations and seated Footwork on the Chair? • Quadruped hip flexion/extension patterns, including Bird Dog, Knee Stretch Variations, etc.? Back—Are the thoracic and lumbar spinal erector muscles overworking during: • Standing (two legs and one leg)? • Pulling straps on reformer? • Hamstring curls on reformer? Does the client over-recruit these muscles when performing spinal extension exercises, such as Swan? Abdominals—In standing posture: • Is pelvis neutral, or anteriorly tilted (with hip flexor, low back gripping), or posteriorly tilted (with abdominals, hip extensors gripping)? • Are lines of tension evident in obliques and rectus abdominis?

Kinesthetic Milestone	Pilates Exercises
Gripping Patterns in Back, Abdominals, and Hips (continued)	Hip Flexors—Does the client exhibit hip flexor tension in: • Thomas Test on the cadillac? • Leg Circles on the mat? Pelvic Floor/Glutes—Does the client squeeze and/or tuck this area during: • Footwork? • A crunch? • Standing one- and two-leg patterns?
Thoracic Mobility Can the client mobilize and/or articulate the thoracic spine while stabilizing the lumbar spine and pelvis during …	• Standing and seated Roll-Down variations (against wall, Spine Stretch Forward, etc.)? • Spring-assisted Roll-Backs? • Lateral flexion patterns (Short Box, Mermaid variations, etc.)? • Spine twists in seated, standing, and quadruped positions, or lunge variations?
Flow Invite the experience of flow into every session. Even the most basic patterns can be explored in a flowing way. Do not expect perfection, but at every moment know that fluidity is the goal and adjust the speed, load, and range of motion to find the "sweet spot" where easing can occur.	• Is the movement jerky, bulging, collapsed, or overly braced?

Exercises for Exploring Kinesthetic Milestones

When you put together your Pilates class or private session, choose one or two kinesthetic milestones and organize your exercise choices and cueing around these, to provide a sense of coherency and direction to the session.

Below are some standard Pilates and therapeutic exercises that feature basic movement patterns that are ideal for conveying the kinesthetic milestones. It is important to reinforce this awareness in a variety of planes of gravity so that the body and brain are prepared for handling the varied environments outside of the studio; the exercises therefore include supine, prone, quadruped, side-lying, seated, and standing positions. The instructions for an exercise will vary depending on which kinesthetic milestone is being emphasized. Change the cueing (using your own language and suggestions from the table in the preceding section) to emphasize different milestones.

Leg Slides

Begin on the back with feet flat, knees bent, and hands on the stomach to feel core engagement. Slide one leg long down the mat and then draw it back up. Repeat on the other side.

On the reformer (one or two springs): Lying supine on the reformer with one foot on the footbar and the other in table top position, slowly press the carriage out and bring it back in, lightly resisting the pull of the spring. Repeat several times with one leg and then switch to the other leg.

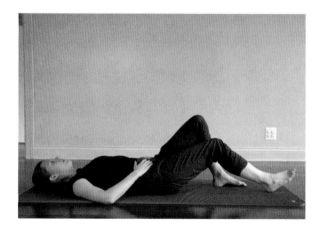

Footwork (three heavy springs)
Leg Springs (one heavy spring, one medium)

On the reformer: Lie supine on the reformer (neutral pelvis) with both feet on the footbar (or Leg Springs). On the footbar, positions can include parallel (heels, arches, and between the balls of the feet and the toes); in Footwork *and* Leg Springs, feet can be turned out (heels together, toes apart), in wide squat position, or other variations. Slowly press the carriage out and bring it back in, lightly resisting the pull of the spring. Repeat several times. In Leg Springs, try making double circles, rectangles, and/or triangles in each direction.

Footwork

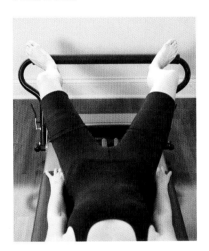 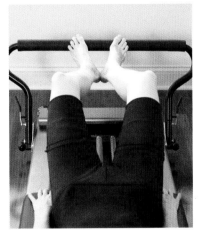 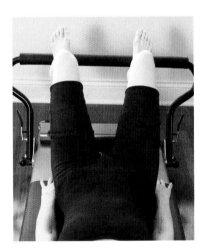

Leg Springs

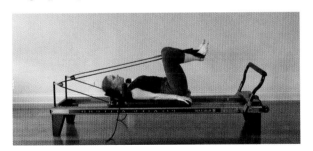 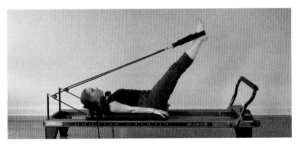

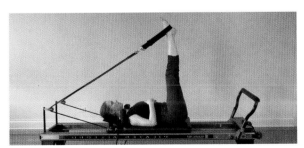

Marching and Lower Lift Variations

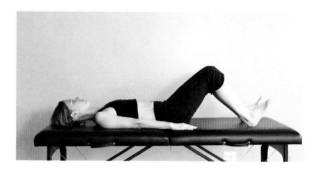

- First progression—Begin in the supine, bent-knee, neutral-pelvis position. Lift one knee up above the hip, maintaining lower-rib contact with the mat. Return to start position and alternate sides.

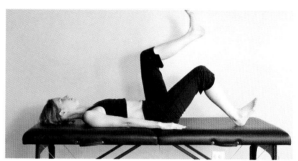

- Second progression—Begin in table top position (feet lifted off the floor, knees above the hips). Drop one foot to the floor, maintaining a 90-degree angle at the knee, and lower-rib contact with the mat. Lift the foot back to the start position. Alternate sides.

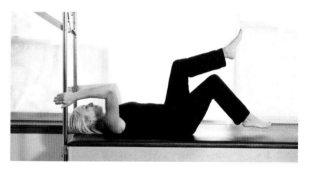

- Third progression—Lower Lift (modified variation). Both knees lower any amount towards the floor, maintaining lower-rib contact with the mat and front rib integration. Be sure the pelvis remains stable to avoid straining the low back. Lift back to the start position and repeat.

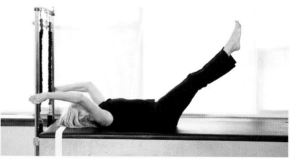

- Fourth progression—Lower Lift (full variation). Both legs are fully extended and lower together any amount towards the floor, maintaining lower-rib contact with the mat and front rib integration. Be sure that the pelvis remains stable to avoid straining the low back. Return to the start position and repeat.

Chest Lift/Crunch

Assume supine position with pelvis in neutral. Place hands lightly behind the head, providing some support for the neck. On the exhale, lift the head and chest; inhale to lower. Maintain a neutral pelvis throughout the movement. Lift the lower abdominals and keep a full posterolateral expansion of the ribcage to prevent excessive downward intra-abdominal pressure on the pelvic floor. To activate the upper abdominals, slide the lower tip of the sternum towards the pubic bone and reach the tip of the nose towards the navel.

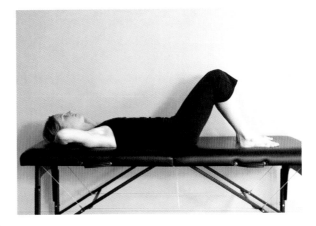

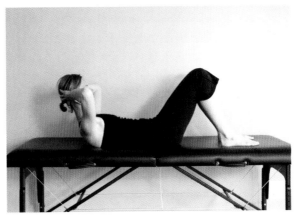

Bridging Variations: Mat or Reformer

On the mat: Lie supine, feet flat and knees bent. Roll up bone by bone, using your X-ray vision to feel each vertebra articulate through the movement. Return to the mat in the same way. Repeat, always concentrating on the movement of each individual bone.

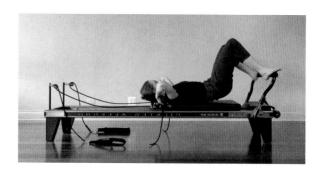

On the reformer: Lower the headrest and attach two to five springs (start heavier and reduce tension to increase the challenge).

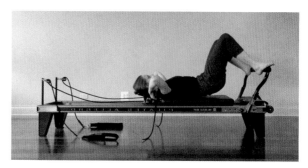

- Lying on your back, place the heels of the feet wide on the footbar. (Footbar is on the top setting.)
- Roll up (starting with the hips) to the lowest rib. In other words, the lowest rib should be touching the mat but the hips should be lifted.

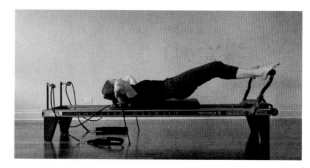

- Breathe into this band across the low back ribs (the thoracolumbar junction) and feel the ribs expand into the mat. Softly thread the front ribs together, as though tying a corset.
- Press through the feet and extend the legs, moving the carriage away from the footbar, breathing naturally. Try not to allow the low back ribs to lose contact with the mat.
- Return the carriage to the start position, taking care to maintain the position of the spine (hips lifted, low back ribs touching the mat).
- Continue this movement, in and out, concentrating on breathing into the low back ribs and threading the front ribs.

Swan

Lying prone, bend your elbows and stack your hands to make a pillow for your forehead. Press your pubic bone into the mat and gently scoop the abdominals.

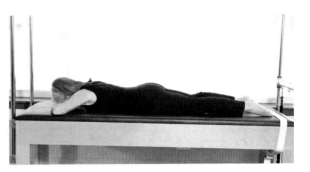

- To begin, lift the head and shoulders only, rolling just to the point where the base of your sternum remains anchored to the mat. Repeat this action, feeling for the upper back muscles while encouraging the low back muscles to remain quiet.

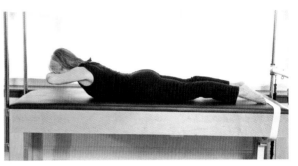

- Once you have found the upper back muscles, increase the difficulty by keeping the hands glued to the forehead and lifting the hands and arms as well.
- Finally, continue to lift the spine higher, always initiating with the upper back muscles and maintaining deep abdominal support to protect the low back. Lift and broaden through the heart and sternum to encourage opening in this area. On the way down, press every backbone forward towards the mat, feeling the articulation of each vertebra.

Knee Stretch Variations

Prep: Set one heavy spring on the reformer. Assume a quadruped position with the feet against the shoulder rests and the forearms on the footbar. For more comfort, you can adjust the footbar to a lower setting and place the short box across it, making sure that it is secure.

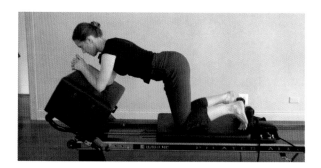

To ensure that clients first learn the difference between pushing the carriage out with their arms (and stabilizing the hips) and pushing out with the legs (and stabilizing the arms), make sure that they have differentiated between these two patterns by practicing them a few times.

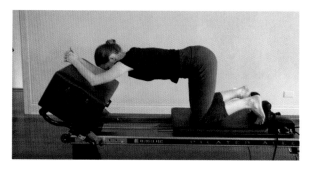

- Inhaling, fill the belly and push the carriage out using only the legs (not the arms).
- Pause. Scoop the belly. (Trainers, you can place your hand on the client's stomach to help them find this scoop.)
- Exhaling, slowly draw the carriage in to the bumper.
- Repeat.
- When you are comfortable with this pattern, speed it up, keeping the low back and pelvis steady.

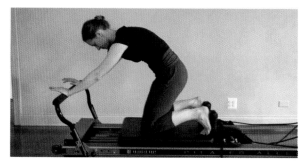

You may then progress to full Knee Stretches (one heavy, one medium spring). Remove the box and lift the footbar. Place the hard part of your palm onto the footbar (thumbs with fingers) and straighten your arms, sitting back onto your heels (variations include flexed or extended spine). Repeat the previous exercise with more natural breathing. The core is gently lifted through the entire movement pattern. Knees move back and forth with increasing speed. The pelvis stays steady in a neutral position (i.e., the low back does not hinge between flexed and extended positions).

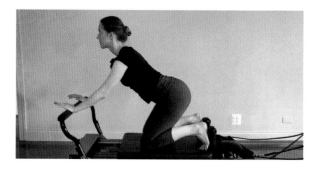

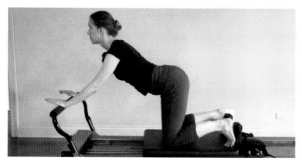

Elephant

Set one heavy and one medium spring on the reformer. Carefully step onto the reformer with hands on the footbar and heels at the shoulder rests like a Downward Dog position in yoga. Thumbs should be with the fingers, and the hard part of the palms should rest on the footbar. Draw the shoulders away from the ears.

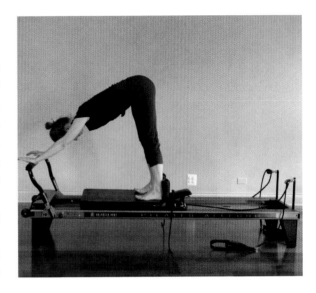

- Inhaling, fill the belly and push the carriage out using only the legs (not the arms).
- Pause. Scoop the belly. (Trainers, you can place your hand on the client's stomach to help them find this scoop.)
- Exhaling, slowly draw the carriage in to the bumper on a three-count.
- Repeat.

Bird Dog

Begin on hands and knees (in quadruped position) with shoulders over wrists, and hips over knees. Activate the deep core and elongate the spine, tail to crown.

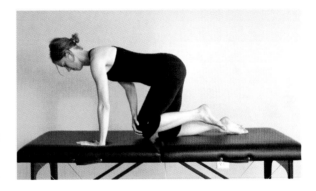

Variation 1: Hover the left hand and the right knee. Change sides. Alternate side to side, working to maintain the stability in the hips and low back.

Variation 2: Extend the left arm and the right leg. Try to maintain a neutral spine and pelvic position. Now bring the hand and knee to meet in front of the navel. Repeat, extending the arm and leg and then touching hand to knee. Do this slowly 6–12 times, and then rest and repeat on the other side.

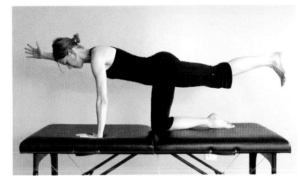

Variation 3: Hover (and/or extend) the *same* side leg and arm in the manner described above.

Variation 4: For a fun challenge, try these variations while kneeling on a foam roller!

Quadruped and Low Lunge Variations

Practice all of these forward flexion and rotation patterns on all fours (or for more of a challenge, bring one foot forward into a low lunge, maintaining a 90-degree angle at each knee and hip).

Cat/Cow: The Cat and Cow Stretch involves alternately rounding, or flexing, the spine (Cat Stretch) and arching, or extending, the spine (Cow Stretch). For variety, rather than just flexing and extending the back in an alternating pattern, work to enhance your brain's mental map of your spine by aiming to articulate one vertebra at a time. If you are in a Cat Stretch, begin by curling your tailbone up to the ceiling and then work your way through each segment of your spine, lastly lifting the neck and then the head. To return to a Cat Stretch, begin again at the tailbone, curling it between the legs, and articulating the backbones slowly to the head.

Rotation: Lift one hand and reach it across the midline of the body (towards the front leg if lunging). With tiny, gentle bounces aimed at the deep rotators of the spine, reach and explore the area between your opposite hand and knee (or hip, if you have stepped your foot forward). Do not stop there. Continue this pulsing reach in the area parallel to the floor above your head and towards your supporting arm.

Practice thoracic extension and rotation patterns in quadruped by rotating one arm away from the midline of the body towards the ceiling and then back to quadruped or lunging.

Practice lateral flexion by rotating away from the midline and then reaching the arm parallel to the floor like a Side-Angle Pose in yoga.

Finally the most complex pattern: Combine the previous two motions (rotation and lateral flexion) into a freestyle swimming pattern. Rotate to the ceiling, then laterally flex with an elongated reach, and then return to the start position, with shoulders squared to the floor. Take care to ensure that the arm motion begins with thoracic rotation, or you will risk injuring the shoulder.

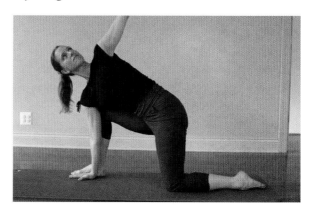

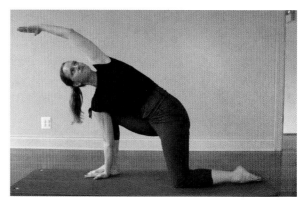

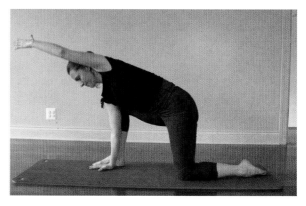

One-Arm Push-Up Variations in Quadruped or Plank on the Wunda/Exo Chair

Set one spring on the chair. In full Plank, kneeling, or with one leg extended, place one hand on the mat and the other on the pedal. Press the pedal to the floor and then carefully return it to the start position, maintaining the torso and pelvis square to the floor the entire time (they will want to rotate towards the pedal). Repeat several times and then change sides.

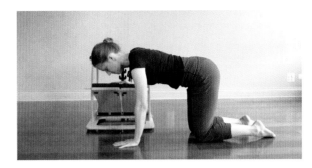

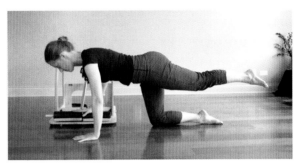

Side-Lying Footwork on the Reformer

Set one or two springs on the reformer. Lie on one side, with the head in the headrest (add a pillow for additional comfort) and hips back at the edge of the carriage. The hips are stacked and the bottom leg is bent in towards the chest. The top foot is on the footbar, with the heel in line with the knee. Do not allow the knee to drop below the level of the top hip. To begin, press the top leg straight, maintaining a long, low spine and a neutral pelvic position. Bending the knee, return to the start position. Repeat several times and then change sides.

For a more challenging variation in side-lying, try this while jumping on the jumpboard or with one foot in a leg spring!

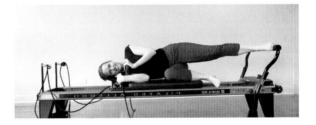

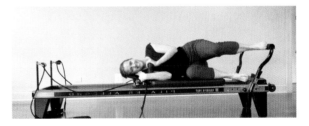

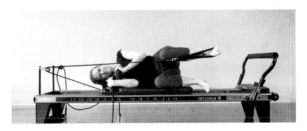

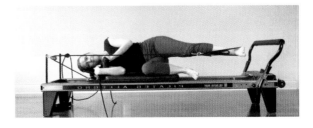

Octopus Tentacles

This exercise can be performed on the mat or on any apparatus, using a spring or a stretch band. Begin in a side-lying position, with hips stacked and pelvis in neutral. Move the leg around in any direction, like the tentacle of an octopus. Feel how this movement emanates from the core. Practice keeping the low back and hips steady during this motion. Practice this in a variety of ways. Explore and strive for ease, applying all the kinesthetic milestones.

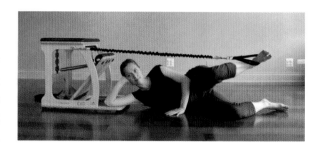

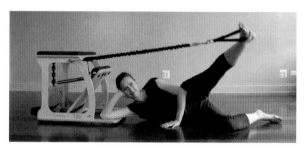

Round Back Variations

Sit on the floor, with the knees bent and feet flat. Lightly hold behind the thighs. Round the spine and gaze towards your navel. Inhale and round the back, lengthening the arms and filling the belly with air. Exhale and return to the starting position, drawing the navel to the spine. Repeat this pattern several times. Now place one hand on the belly and leave the other hand behind the thigh. Repeat the exercise, inhaling on the way back and exhaling forward. Feel the tummy flesh expand beneath your hand as you inhale and pull away from the hand as you exhale. Practice until you feel comfortable with this action. With springs, practice rolling back and up, using the tension of the springs to assist you through the difficult parts. Remember the kinesthetic milestones!

On the short box (see the photo in the next exercise), place both feet under the safety strap. Place both hands on the stomach. Inhale on the way back, filling the belly with air. Exhale on the way forward and feel the belly pull away from the hands. Repeat several times.

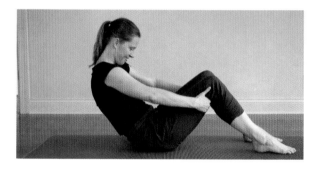

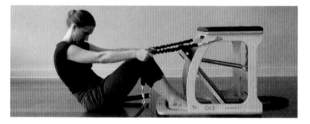

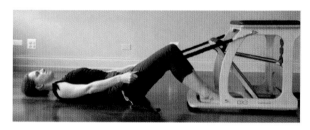

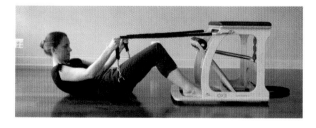

Short Box Series Variations (seated, in kneeling lunge, or in standing lunge)

Short box exercises offer some of the best thoracic mobilization opportunities (e.g., side bends, twist, twist with reach, row the boat). Many of these can also be done in a standing lunge (or Warrior pose, for yogis). Lateral flexion, rotation, flexion, and rolling-up patterns come alive with sensation and challenge when you take into account the principles above. There is no need to stick rigidly to the classical patterns. Get creative in your short box movements.

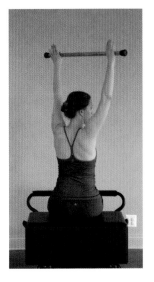
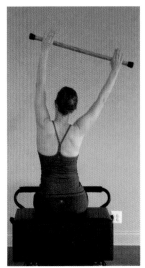

Add forward flexion with rotation (e.g., Saw) with arms out to the side like the letter "T." You can work through the traditional Saw pattern in large sweeping movements (rotate, reach down, roll up, other side). This will work the larger muscle chains of the upper body. Also try inserting tiny bounces at the end range of your forward-rotation-reach. In contrast to the large sweeping motions, this variation helps to awaken and stretch the deep lateral rotators of the spine. Then, in this subtle bouncing manner, explore the entire range between the floor and the ceiling. Notice where you feel restriction.

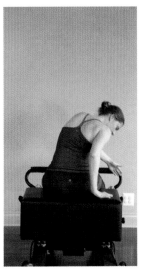
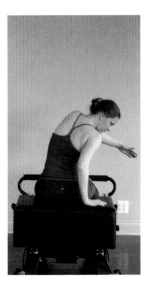

Next, emphasize thoracic extension as you rotate away from the midline. Reach your arms towards the ceiling in a "V" and add tiny bounces. Reach higher and higher as you do this, opening up and bending back only through the heart area (lumbar spine is long and TLJ is stable).

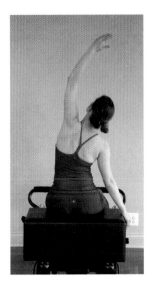
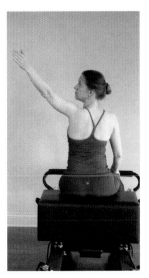

Row the boat forward over your legs, then to the left, and then to the right. Go where you need the stretch, and when you find a restriction, stay and breathe deeply, inflating your ribs directly into that area. For additional proprioceptive challenge, try performing these variations in a kneeling, or standing, lunge position!

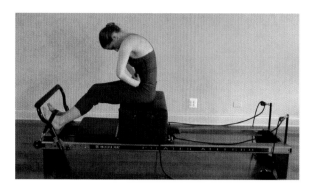

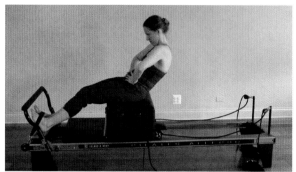

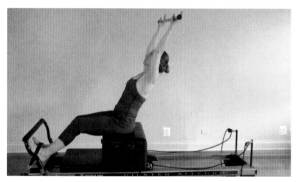

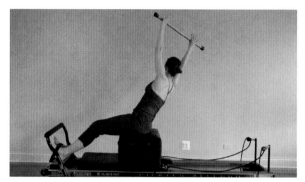

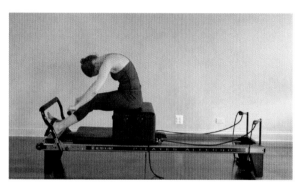

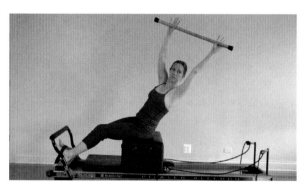

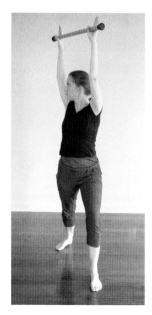

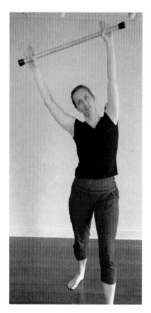

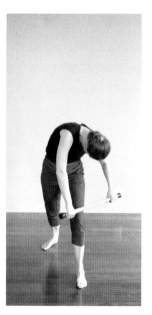

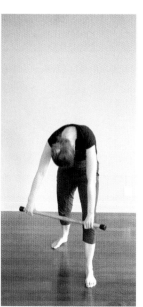

Stomach Massage Variations

On the reformer: Set one to four springs. Sit on the carriage, with the feet on the footbar (traditionally, heels together and toes apart, but modify as appropriate), pelvis in neutral, and spine as long as possible. (To avoid sliding, you may need to sit on a sticky pad.) To assist with axial elongation, you may initially choose to use the arms to help lift the spine by pushing into the carriage or reaching behind to the shoulder rests. (More advanced variations involve reaching the arms ahead or up to the ceiling.) To begin, extend the legs, pressing the carriage away from the footbar. Growing ever longer through the spine, return to the start position and repeat.

For a more forgiving variation, reduce the number of springs and lower the feet to the lower sides of the footbar or onto the platform.

For a more challenging variation, add thoracic rotation on the leg extension.

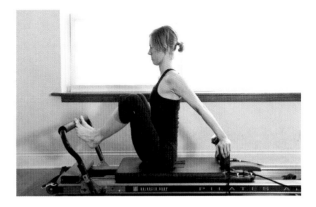

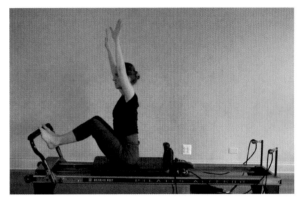

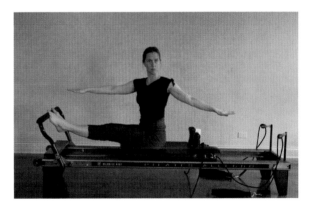

Mermaid Variations: Reformer or Mat

Mermaid is traditionally performed in a "Z-sit" position, with one hand (the hand on the side of the bent knees) on the floor or the footbar of the reformer (one spring). On an inhale the opposite hand reaches up to the ceiling over to the side, as the spine laterally flexes towards the anchored hand. On the reformer, the carriage slides away from the footbar. To complete the breath cycle, the spine returns to its upright position. Repeat.

There are many ways to add a flowing dynamic to this exercise. One fun variation is to try using a furniture slider (with both hands on the slider) to "scrub" the floor. Move with a combination of fluidity and gentle bouncing, stretching and articulating the spine in a way that feels good. Move to the front and sides, breathing and working through the areas that feel stuck.

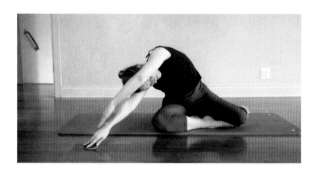
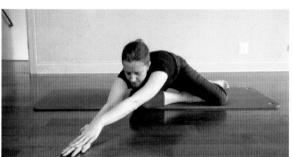

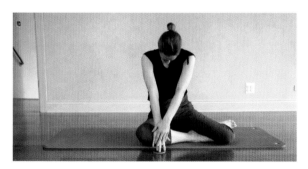
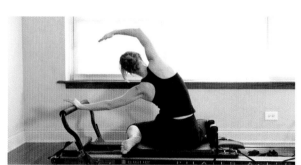

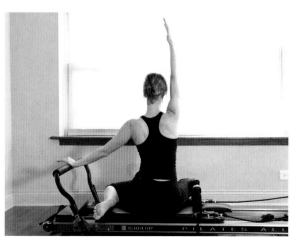
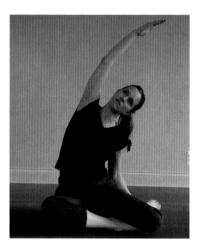

Seated Knee Extension and Hip Flexion

Seated in a chair, or on the short box, sit up tall, with a neutral pelvis. Lift one bent knee and hold under the thigh. Practice lengthening and bending the leg while maintaining a long spine. (Trainers, note where the spine goes into flexion and encourage the client to lengthen in this area.)

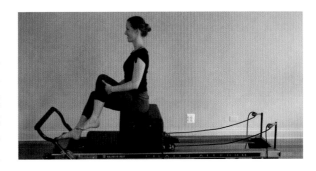

Next, try letting go of the leg and holding it up a few inches off the ground while maintaining a long spine. For an additional challenge, press down into the top of the leg as the leg presses up into the palms of your hands. Continue to elongate the low spine against the compressive force of your trunk and hip flexor contraction.

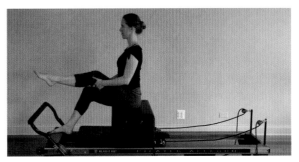

Spine Stretch Forward: Mat or Reformer

On the mat: Sit on the floor, with legs extended in front. Feel free to elevate the hips with a bolster and bend the knees, as needed, to ensure a neutral pelvis and a long (not flexed) low spine. Draw the abdominals in and elongate the spine. Maintaining this lift in the low spine, begin to articulate from the head to the mid-back, flexing one bone at a time. To return to seated, articulate the spine to the start position, using the muscles of the upper back. Repeat.

On the reformer: Your reformer must be elevated on legs to perform this variation of the exercise. Set one spring on the reformer. Sit on the floor in "the well" of the reformer (the space between the carriage and the back frame), with the legs extended in front underneath the carriage. Elevate the hips with a bolster and bend the knees as needed to ensure a neutral pelvis and a long (not flexed) low spine. Sit at a distance such that there is some tension in the spring when the hard parts of the palms of the hands are hooked around the shoulder rests. To begin, draw the abdominals in and

elongate the spine. Maintaining this lift in the low spine, begin to articulate from the head to the mid-back, flexing one bone at a time. Allow the tension on the spring to pull you forward as you gently resist flexing the low spine with a sense of elongation. Breathe into any areas of tightness. To return to seated, articulate the spine to the start position, using the muscles of the upper back. Repeat.

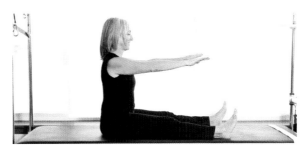

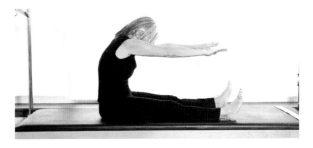

One-Leg Press on the Chair

Set one spring on the chair. Stand facing the chair, femur-length away from the pedal. Lift one foot and place it on the pedal. Elongate the spine and press the pedal down towards the floor (not all the way). Return the pedal to the top, with control. Repeat several times then change sides.

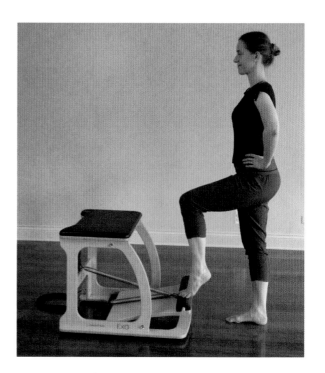

For added proprioceptive challenge, bring the hands together and twist the torso reaching the arms to the right as the foot presses the pedal down. Bend the elbows and rotate center while controlling the upward movement of the pedal. Repeat the same motion to the left. Create variation and challenge by adding other movements while pressing the pedal down (e.g. thoracic flexion/extension, lateral spinal flexion, or hinging at the hips with a long straight spine paying special attention to lumbar stability).

For added challenge, when you press down on the pedal:
• Try laterally flexing the thoracic spine side to side with arms overhead.
• Try rotating the thoracic spine and adding an arm reach.
• Bow forward, taking care to stabilize all the vertebral joints, especially the lumbar joints (T12-S1).
• To strengthen the muscles that support the arch of the foot, combine the bowing motion with a downward reach to one side and then the other.

Going Up Front on the Chair

Set two strong springs on the chair. To mount the chair, place both hands on either side of the "seat" of the chair. Place one foot on the pedal and lean your body weight into the pedal to lower it to the ground. Step the other foot onto the pedal. Choose one foot and place it up onto the seat of the chair, with the toes towards the back edge. Stand all the way up onto that leg, and adjust the back foot on the pedal. Lower down until your stationary leg is at a 90-degree angle in the hip and knee. Anchor the tripod of the foot and press back up to the top. Repeat several times and then change sides.

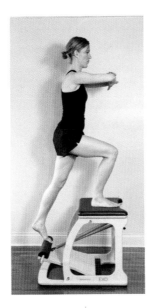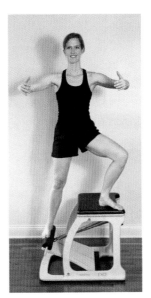

Note: To begin, you may want to practice this on the high chair or with the wunda/exo chair pressed against a wall to provide more support.

(Also pictured, Going Up Side Variation)

Lunge Variations on the Reformer

Set one heavy spring on the reformer. Standing on the left side of the reformer carriage, place the sole of the right foot against the shoulder rest, knee resting on the carriage and toes curled in extension. Place the left foot near the leg of the reformer and hands (or fingertips) on the footbar. Press the right leg back, engaging the hip extensor muscles and maintaining a neutral pelvis (to avoid anterior femoral glide). Feel the stretch to the front of the right hip as the left glute and quadriceps muscles work isometrically to stabilize the leg. Continue this movement several times and then repeat on the other side.

To advance the exercise:
• Lift the back knee and keep it lifted as the leg and carriage move forward and back.
• Remove the hands from the footbar.
• Add thoracic rotation. As the right leg moves back, rotate the ribcage to the left. As the right leg moves forward, rotate the ribcage.
•Add thoracic lateral flexion with arms overhead.
• Bow forward as the leg pushes back (taking care to stabilize the joints of the lumbar spine), using the glutes and hamstrings of the stationary leg to return to an upright position.

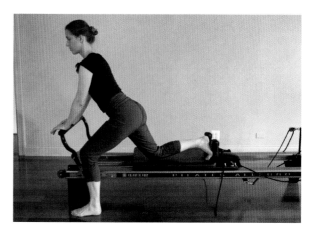

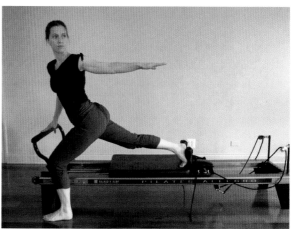

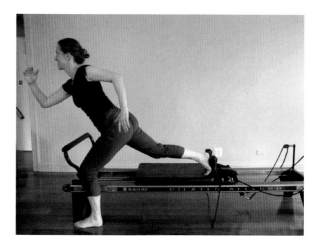

Glossary

Activation
Techniques to stimulate the proprioceptive (sensory) system to increase the strength or responsiveness of a muscle or groups of muscles. In other words, these are strategies to turn a muscle "on" when it has become inhibited or turned "off" secondary to trauma, inflammation, and/or disuse. Techniques for activation include visualization (to get the central nervous system to connect to the muscle), isometric contractions (to stabilize a joint position and turn on muscles around the joint), palpation of musculofascial attachments, ligaments, skin, and/or joint capsule (to stimulate the proprioceptors), and breathing (to activate the diaphragm and other muscles of the deep myofascial system).

Autonomic Nervous System
A division of the peripheral nervous system that influences function of the internal organs, including heart and respiratory rates as well as the digestive and urogenital systems. The ANS is subdivided into the sympathetic (fight-or-flight) and parasympathetic (rest-and-digest) nervous systems.

Axis of Rotation
The imaginary central point or line through a joint around which the joint rotates. Imagine the axis of rotation as the axis around which the tire spins on a car. In the body, the axis is determined by the shape of the joints as well as by the soft tissue structures (joint capsule and ligaments) that surround the joint. Maintaining an ideal axis of rotation is a requirement of smooth, coordinated movement and is reliant upon optimal control of motion.

Bracing Strategy
Contraction of the muscles surrounding a joint to improve stabilization. For example, co-contraction of the abdominals and erector spinae muscles around the trunk and spine provide core stabilization. This is an effective strategy for stabilizing an isometric position, but may become detrimental if maintained for long periods of time and/or it is the individual's primary stabilization strategy.

Breath Activation Strategy
Utilizing three-dimensional breathing and activation of the deep myofascial system to develop an optimal strategy of core stabilization. The Breath Activation Strategy helps develop coordination between breathing and activation of the deep myofascial system and should be established prior to instituting higher-level Pilates exercises.

Centering
Placing the core of the body in the most optimal position for performing exercises. For many exercise patterns, this will include achieving neutral alignment of the head, thorax, lumbar spine, and pelvis prior to, and returning from, a specific movement pattern.

Central Nervous System
The part of the nervous system that includes the brain and spinal cord and governs all activity within the body.

Co-activation
A contraction of the muscles surrounding a joint or region of the body to maintain an optimum axis of rotation and joint control, whether in a static position or moving. In others words, there are different muscles working together at the same time to provide support for the joint and allow it to stabilize and move without losing its optimal position.

Concentric Contraction
A muscle contraction in which the attachments of the muscle are getting closer together in order to move or accelerate the bone to which the muscle is attached. Lifting a weight or body region and/or acceleration of the body generally involve concentric contractions.

Control
Conscious or subconscious ability to create smooth, coordinated posture and movement. Control is a prerequisite to producing smooth, coordinated movement without the need to compensate to achieve stability and can be developed with the application of the Pilates principles.

Core Stabilization
A strategy for aligning and controlling the body so that the joints are appropriately positioned and the myofascial system is able to accommodate the demands of the task in an efficient manner. Core stabilization must be maintained not only in the static position but also during a dynamic movement; however, the strategy utilized—the amount of effort—will vary depending on the demands of the task.

Corrective Exercise
Exercise designed to specifically address postural alterations, non-optimal stabilization strategies, and/or non-optimal movement patterns. In other words, these are exercises or strategies created to achieve optimal posture and movement while placing the least amount of stress on the muscles and joints so that the likelihood of injury is reduced.

Eccentric Contraction
A muscle contraction in which the muscle attachments are getting further apart in order to decelerate or slow down a movement. Lowering a weight or body region and/or slowing down one's momentum generally involve eccentric contractions.

Fascia
A dense connective tissue invested into virtually every structure throughout the body. Fascia contains contractile and sensory elements, thereby allowing it to assist posture, stabilization, and movement. The myofascial system (connection of the muscle and fascial systems) provides the support for posture and movement.

Feed-Forward Mechanism
Anticipatory pre-contraction of certain muscles (generally the one-joint muscles) milliseconds before a prime movement occurs in order to stabilize joint structures. For example, the transversus abdominis and pelvic floor pre-activate prior to the initiation of limb motion in individuals without pain or trauma, as demonstrated in the research.

Flexion Intolerance

A low tolerance for flexion positions. Generally these individuals will experience back discomfort and/or muscle inhibition during positions of spinal flexion (sitting, bending forward, performing flexion-based exercises such as Crunches, Roll-Ups, Hundreds).

Force Closure

Contraction of the myofascial system to provide joint stability. Optimal force closure provides the stabilization and control required for posture and movement.

Form Closure

The inherent shape of the joints and surrounding ligaments and joint capsule that provides joint stability. For example, the sacroiliac joint has high form closure, because the wedge-shaped sacrum is held between the two innominate bones and there are projections on the articulating surfaces. In contrast, the glenohumeral joint of the shoulder has low form closure, as it is a ball and socket joint and the humeral head is significantly larger than the articulating surface on the glenoid fossa. Regardless of the level of form closure, all joints rely upon the myofascial system or force closure for stability.

Gripping

Over-contraction of the myofascial system to provide joint stabilization and/or control. Gripping usually occurs either consciously (trying to squeeze muscles because more contraction is often viewed as being better) or subconsciously (reflexive contraction secondary to muscle inhibition) after surgery or other trauma, or during inflammation. Individuals will generally experience chronic tightness and/or trigger points in the region(s) of the body where they are gripping.

Inhibition

The desensitization or lack of optimal neurological input into the myofascial system. Inhibition usually occurs secondary to trauma, surgery, and/or inflammation and results in a weakened muscle response. Inhibited muscles must be activated and then integrated into the appropriate movement patterns.

Integration

Optimal coordination of alignment, breathing, and control while performing the fundamental Pilates patterns.

Intra-abdominal Pressure

Pressure generated within the abdominal cavity as a result of contraction of the diaphragm, abdominals, intercostals, and other muscles of respiration. Intra-abdominal pressure aids stabilization and decompression of (i.e., less compression of, or stress upon) the trunk, spine, and pelvis.

Isometric Contraction

A muscle contraction where there is no net change in the length of the muscle. These types of contraction are used to stabilize a joint or body position, as well as occurring during the transition between eccentric and concentric contractions.

Kinesthesia

The process of developing awareness and physical dexterity in areas of the body. Kinesthesia is one of the vital components in improving posture and movement, as the individual must often increase their kinesthesia or awareness of current habits in order to adopt and/or develop more ideal ones.

Myofascial Lines/Chains

Groups of myofascia of the deep and superficial myofascial systems which are anatomically and functionally linked together and contribute to various positions and movements.

Myofascial System

The system comprised of the skeletal muscles and their investing fascia. It is subdivided into the deep myofascial system (deep muscles and their fascia that attach directly to the joints) and superficial myofascial system (superficial muscles and their fascia), which are arranged in myofascial lines or chains.

Neuroplasticity

The ability of the brain to change and adapt its synapses and neural networks via different kinds of stimulation, including (but not limited to) physical activity, mental stimuli, environment, education, and pain. The act of being aware, using imagery and conscious control during exercises, is a way of improving neuroplasticity of the brain.

Neutral Alignment

The position in which there is ideal alignment of posture and movement that benefits loading of the joints while minimizing wear and tear of the soft tissue and bony structures. Helping individuals develop awareness and control of neutral alignment of the core is one of the early and important components in developing ideal posture and movement.

Peripheral Nervous System

The portion of the nervous system that includes the cranial and spinal nerves. The peripheral nervous system receives and transmits messages between the body and the central nervous system.

Proprioception

The nervous system's ability to receive information from the muscles, fascia, ligaments, and joint receptors, as well as from the visual and vestibular systems, in order to sense and adjust posture and movement.

Rigidity

Stiffness and loss of mobility in a joint or region of the body due to over-activation of the myofascial system. Rigidity often limits range and ease of motion. When it occurs around the thorax, rigidity will limit optimal three-dimensional breathing and over time will create excessive joint tension.

Somatic Nervous System

The portion of the nervous system responsible for voluntary control of skeletal muscles. The somatic nervous system includes both cranial and spinal nerves.

Synergist Dominance
The assumption by the synergists of the role of primary stabilizers or movers in the presence of muscle or joint inhibition. In other words, muscles that are designed to assist in a motion take the role of dominant muscle in the action. For example, inhibition of the gluteus maximus can cause the hamstrings to become the prime movers of hip extension. Muscles that become synergistically dominant are often those that an individual tends to grip with and the reason why chronic tightness develops in these regions.

Tensegrity
The ability of the myofascial system to stabilize the body via tension and a "floating" compression to allow stresses to be spread out through the body as opposed to being centered in any one area. Tensegrity enables elongation and suspension of the body instead of resorting to over-compression for stability and movement.

Thoracopelvic Canister
The collective regions of the thoracic spine, ribcage, lumbar spine, and pelvis. Also referred to as the core.

Three-Dimensional Breathing
The ability to utilize the entire thoracic, abdominal, and pelvic cavities so that during the breath cycle these regions expand and relax in three dimensions—superiorly–inferiorly (top to bottom), laterally (side to side), and anteroposteriorly (front to back).

Bibliography

Baniel, A. 2009. *Move into Life: The Nine Essentials for Lifelong Vitality*. Random House, Inc.: New York, NY.

Baniel, A. 2012. *Kids Beyond Limits*. Perigee: New York, NY.

Barker, K.L., Shamley, D.R., and Jackson, D. 2000. Changes in the cross-sectional area of multifidus and psoas in patients with unilateral back pain: The relationship to pain and disability. *Clinical Journal of Sport Medicine* 10(4), 239–244.

Black, J. 2013. *Making the American Body*. University of Nebraska Press: Lincoln, NE.

Butler, D. and Moseley, L. 2013. *Explain Pain*. Noigroup Publications: Adelaide, Australia.

Calais-Germain, B. 2008. *No Risk Abs*. Healing Arts Press: Rochester, VT.

Calais-Germain, B. and Raison, B. 2010. No *Risk Pilates*. Healing Arts Press: Rochester, VT.

Chaitow, L., Bradley, D., and Gilbert, C. 2014. *Recognizing and Treating Breathing Disorders*, 2nd edn. Churchill Livingston: Edinburgh.

Chaitow, L., Findley, T.W., and Schleip, R. 2012. *Fascia Research III*. Kiener: Munich.

Clippinger, K. 2007. *Dance Anatomy and Kinesiology. Human Kinetics*: Champaign, IL.

Cohen, R. 2010. Introduction to Reflex Locomotion According to Vojta (Course handouts). Philadelphia, PA.

Davies, C. 2004. *The Trigger Point Therapy Workbook*, 2nd edn. New Harbinger Publications: Oakland, CA.

Eherer, A.J., Netolitzky, F., Hogenauer, C., Puschnig, G., Hinterleitner, T.A., Scheidl, S., Kraxner, W., Kreis, G.J., and Hoffmann, K.M. 2012. Positive effect of abdominal breathing exercise on gastroesophageal reflux disease: A randomized, controlled study. *American Journal of Gastroenterology* 107(3), 372–378.

Eunyoung, K. and Lee, H. 2013. The effects of deep abdominal muscle strengthening exercises on respiratory function and lumbar stability. *Journal of Physical Therapy Science* 25, 663–665.

Gibbons, S. 2005. Assessment and rehabilitation of the stability function of the psoas major and the deep sacral gluteus maximus muscles. Kinetic Control: Ludlow, UK.

Gibbons, S.G.T. and Comerford, M.J. 2001a. Strength versus stability—Part 1: Concepts and terms. *Orthopaedic Division Review*, Mar/Apr, 21–27.

Gibbons, S.G.T. and Comerford, M.J. 2001b. Strength versus stability—Part 2: Limitations and benefits. *Orthopaedic Division Review*, Mar/Apr, 28–33.

Gibbons, S.G.T., Comerford, M.J., and Emerson, P.L. 2002. Rehabilitation of the stability function of psoas major. *Orthopaedic Division Review*, Jan/Feb, 9–16.

Gibbons, S.G.T., Mottram, S.L., Comerford, M.J., and Phty, B. 2001. Stability and movement dysfunction related to the elbow and forearm. *Orthopaedic Division Review*, Sep/Oct, 15–33.

Grimaldi, A., Richardson, C.A., Stanton, W.R., Durbridge, G.L., Donnelly, W.J., and Hides, J.A. 2009. The association between degenerative hip joint pathology and size of the gluteus medius, gluteus minimus and piriformis. *Manual Therapy* 14(6), 605–610.

Guimberteau, J-C. 2012. *Skins, Scars, and Stiffness* [DVD]. Endo Vivo Productions: Pessac, France www.endovivo.com.

Hagins, M., Pietrek MD, M., Sheikhzadeh, A., Nordin, M., and Axen, K. 2004. The effects of breath control on intra-abdominal pressure during lifting tasks. *Spine* 29(4), 464–469.

Hodges, P.W. and Gandevia, S.C. 2000. Changes in intra-abdominal pressure during postural and respiratory activation of the human diaphragm. *Journal of Applied Physiology* 89(3), 967–76.

Hodges, P.W., Heijnen, I., and Gandevia, S.C. 2001. Postural activity of the diaphragm is reduced in humans when respiratory demand increases. *Journal of Physiology* 537(3), 999–1008.

Holubcova Z. 2013. Dynamic neuromuscular stabilization: Exercise strategies (Course handouts). Chicago, IL.

Hu, H., Meijer, O.G., van Dieen, J.H., Hodges, P.W., Bruijn, S.M., Strijers, R.L., Prabath, W.B.N., van Royen, B.J., Wu, W.H., and Xia, C. 2011. Is the psoas a hip flexor in the active straight leg raise? *European Spine Journal* 20(5), 759–765.

Hulme, J.A. 2008. Beyond Kegels: *Bladder Health and the Pelvic Muscle Force Field*. The Prometheus Group: Chicago, IL.

Jacobs, J.V., Henry, S.M., Jones, S.L., Hitt, J.R., and Bunn, J.Y. 2011. A history of low back pain associates with altered electromyographic activation patterns in response to perturbations of standing balance. *Journal of Neurophysiology* 106(5), 2506–2514.

Koch, L. 2012. *The Psoas Book*. Guinea Pig Publications: Felton, CA.

Kolář, P. et al. 2013. *Clinical Rehabilitation*. Kobesová Alena: Prague.

Kolář, P., Kobesová, A., and Holubcova, Z. 2009. Dynamic neuromuscular stabilization: A developmental kinesiology approach (Course handouts). Rehabilitation Institute of Chicago: Chicago, IL.

Kolář, P., Holubcova, Z., Frank, C., Liebenson, C., and Kobesová, A. 2009. Exercise and the athlete: Reflexive, rudimentary and fundamental strategies (Course handouts). International Society of Clinical Rehabilitation Specialists: Chicago, IL.

Lee, D. 2003. *The Thorax: An Integrated Approach*. 2nd edn. Diane G. Lee Physiotherapist Corp: White Rock, BC.

Lee, D. 2011. *The Pelvic Girdle: An Approach to the Examination and Treatment of the Lumbopelvic-hip Region*, 4th edn. Churchill Livingstone: Edinburgh.

Lee, D. and Lee, L.J. 2013. *Treating the Whole Person with The Integrated Systems Model* (Discover Physio Course handouts). Vancouver, BC.

Massery, M. 2006. The patient with multi-system impairments affecting breathing mechanics and motor control. In: Frownfelter D. and Dean, E. (eds), *Cardiovascular and Pulmonary Physical Therapy Evidence and Practice*, 4th edn. Mosby & Elsevier Health Sciences: St. Louis, MO, Chapter 39, 695–717.

Massery, M. 2009. If you can't breathe, you can't function— Integrating the pulmonary, neuromuscular, and musculoskeletal systems in pediatric populations (Course handouts). Pathways Center: Glenview, IL.

Massery, M., Hagins, M., Stafford, R., Moerchen, V., and Hodges, P.W. 2013. The effect of airway control by glottal structures on postural stability. *Journal of Applied Physiology* 115(4), 483–490.

Massey, P. 2009. *The Anatomy of Pilates*. Lotus Publishing: Nutbourne, UK.

McGill, S. 2004. *Ultimate Back Fitness and Performance*. Wabuno: Waterloo, ON.

McGill, S. 2007. *Low Back Disorders: Evidence-Based Prevention and Rehabilitation*, 2nd edn. Human Kinetics: Champaign, IL.

Muller, D. and Schliep, R. 2011. Fascial fitness: Fascia oriented training for bodywork and movement therapies. *IASI Yearbook 2011*. IASI: Raleigh, NC, 68–77.

Myers, T.W. 2011. Fascial fitness: Training in the neuromyofascial web. IDEA Fitness Journal, April www.ideafit.com.

Myers, T.W. 2014. *Anatomy Trains: Myofascial Meridians for Manual and Movement Therapists*, 3rd edn. Churchill Livingston: Edinburgh.

Nyggard, I.E., Thompson, F.L., Svengalis, S.L., and Albright, J.P. 1994. Urinary incontinence in elite nulliparous athletes. *Obstetrics and Gynecology* 84(2), 183–187.

O'Dwyer, M. 2008. *My Pelvic Flaw*. Redsock Publishing: Buderim, Australia.

Osar, E. 2012. *Corrective Exercise Solutions to Common Hip and Shoulder Dysfunction*. Lotus Publishing: Chichester, UK.

Osar, E. 2014. Integrative movement specialists certification (Course handouts). Chicago, IL.

Paoletti, S. 2006. *The Fascia*. Eastland Press Inc.: Seattle, WA.

Patel, A.V., Bernstein L., Deka, A., Feigelson, H.S., Campbell, P.T., Gapstur, S.M., Colditz, G.A., and Thun, M.J. 2010. Leisure time spent sitting in relation to total mortality in a prospective cohort of US adults. *American Journal of Epidemiology* 172(4), 419–429.

Radebold, A., Cholewicki, J., Polzhofer, G.K., and Greene, H.S. 2001. Impaired postural control of the lumbar spine is associated with delayed muscle response times in patients with chronic idiopathic low back pain. *Spine* 26(7), 724–730.

Richardson, C., Hides, J., and Hodges, P.W. 2004. Therapeutic Exercise for Lumbopelvic Stabilization: *A Motor Control Approach for the Treatment and Prevention of Low Back Pain*, 2nd edn. Churchill Livingstone: Edinburgh.

Sahrmann, S. 2002. *Diagnosis and Treatment of Movement Impairment Syndromes*. Mosby: St. Louis, MO.

Sapsford, R.R., Richard, C.A., Maher, C.F., and Hodges, P.W. 2008. Pelvic floor muscle activity in different sitting postures in continent and incontinent women. *Archives of Physical Medicine and Rehabilitation* 89(9), 1741–1747.

Schleip, R. and Klingler, W. 2005. Active fascial contractility: Fascia is able to contract and relax in a smooth muscle-like manner and thereby influence biomechanical behavior. Department of Applied Physiology, Ulm University, Germany www.fasciaresearch.de/2005PosterFreiburg.pdf.

Schleip, R., Klingler, W., and Lehmann-Horn, F. 2004a. Active contraction of the thoracolumbar fascia—Indications of a new factor in low back pain research with implications for manual therapy. *Proc. 5th Interdisciplinary World Congress on Low Back and Pelvic Pain*, Melbourne www.fasciaresearch.de/MelbourneReport.pdf.

Schleip, R., Klingler, W., and Lehmann-Horn, F. 2004b. Active fascial contractility: Fascia may be able to contract in a smooth muscle-like manner and thereby influence musculoskeletal dynamics. *Medical Hypotheses* 65, 273–277.

Schleip, R., Klingler, W., and Lehmann-Horn, F. 2007. Fascia is able to contract in a smooth muscle-like manner and thereby influence musculoskeletal mechanics. *Proc. 5th World Congress of Biomechanics*, Munich.

Schleip, R., Findley, W.T., Chaitow, L., and Huijing, P.A. 2012. *Fascia*. Churchill Livingston Elsevier: New York.

Schleip, R., Naylor, I., Ursu, D., Melzer, W., Zorn, A., Wilke, H-J., Lehmann-Horn, F., and Klingler, W. 2006. Passive muscle stiffness may be influenced by active contractility of intramuscular connective tissue. *Medical Hypotheses* 66, 66–71.

Smith, M., Coppieters, M., and Hodges, P. 2005. Effect of experimentally induced low back pain on postural sway with breathing. *Experimental Brain Research* 166(1), 109–117.

Umphred, D.A. 2007. *Neurological Rehabilitation*, 5th edn. Mosby Elsevier: St. Louis, MO.

Wetzler, G. 2014. The listening connection—Another step to "wow" (Discover Physio Course handouts). Vancouver, BC.

Index

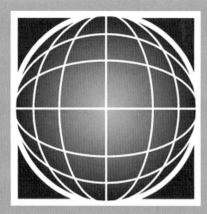
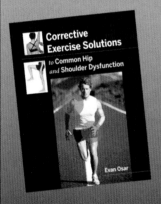
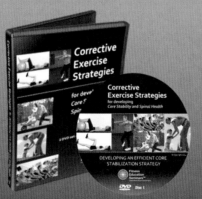
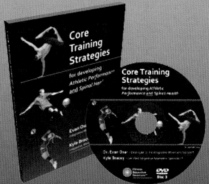
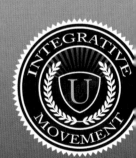
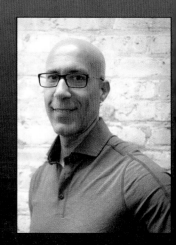